NUMBers

by Kelli Bryant

This publication is non-fiction and based on actual events.

Published in the United States by The JB Group.

Douglasville, GA

ISBN 978-0-578-45094-0

Editor: Carla DuPont

Cover Design: Garrett Myers

PREFACE

There are so many of us who ignore our health. We know something is not right; however, we make every excuse not to go to the doctor. It could be economic circumstances; let's face it, some of us still don't have health insurance. Some of us are just 'too busy.' Some of us are actually afraid of the diagnosis. Whatever the excuse, your health should not be placed on a back burner for later. Later may never come.

The purpose of this book is to bring awareness to Type 2 Diabetes, possible symptoms, and how simple diet choices can help prevent the disease. Family history is also important. This project has been a learning experience. I was encouraged to write *NUMBers* by several friends and colleagues for whom I provided diet and exercise advice. I am proud to say the advice did help them to gain control of their numbers. If you are wondering about the title, NUMB is capitalized because it is a symptom of diabetes. I have experienced NUMBness in the tips of my fingers and in the area between my thumb and pointer finger in my right hand. I have to admit that symptom scared me.

Diabetes is a scary disease to have. If you are not careful, you can experience loss of sight, amputation of limbs, increased risk of cardiovascular events such as heart attacks and strokes, as well as increased damage to other organs such as the kidneys and liver. Many health issues are related to diabetes.

I want to use my experience to help others and possibly contribute to the number of diabetic cases decreasing. It only takes one person to start a trend. I hope you, who are reading these pages, are educated and enjoy the recipe ideas provided in this first volume.

ACKNOWLEDGEMENTS

This publication is non-fiction and based on actual events. Very special thanks to my mother, Darrylyn Blincoe, Dennis Scoggins, Carla DuPont, Yahaira Ledgister, Jameun Bryant, James Bryant III, Jaelun Bryant, Latasha Bryant, Angee Coman Scott, Paula Dockery, Shon Ballard, and Marlene Baez.

This project would not have been possible without the Grace of God.

NUMBers

NUMBers...an Intro

I knew something was going on with my body, but I did not know what it was. My sons and I were on our way back from Blue Springs, Missouri where we celebrated Thanksgiving with new found family.

The year 2015 was full of firsts for us. The highlight of the year was that I was blessed to finally meet family from my father's side whom I had never met. Thanksgiving was the first time I had ever driven from Georgia to Missouri. Two weeks before our journey, I began to experience an extreme thirst that I could not quench. Therefore, I made excessive trips to the restroom. My urine was clear with a slight hint of yellow. One morning, the area between my thumb and pointer finger went numb. I researched these symptoms and diabetes was a possibility.

Since I did not have a primary care physician, I searched for one close. I was able to schedule an appointment for the week of Thanksgiving. I went to my appointment and they scheduled me for labs for the next morning. The morning of Tuesday, November 24, 2015, I went to my lab appointment and afterwards prepared for my 12-hour journey to Missouri for the holiday.

The drive was rough. Remember, I had a thirst issue, and had not yet fully experienced the new symptoms I was about to undergo nor did I know how to handle them. That meant we made more stops than usual for bathroom breaks. My sons were 13, 18, and 19. My 18 and 19-year-old sons had very little driving experience at the time, so I drove the entire way. We made the trip in a little over 15 hours. By the time we made it to my sister's house, I was exhausted. My eyes were so red.

We spent Thanksgiving Day meeting new relatives and enjoying the comradery of the cooked-from-scratch holiday dishes, family conversation, card games, and laughs from memories of holidays past. No dish was off limits. However, I could have killed to have a gallon of every drink in town to quench that damning thirst. I started flushing my system with water instead of the sugary drinks I craved and my thirst seemed to slightly subside.

We began our journey back to Georgia around 11:30 a.m. Central on Sunday, November 29, 2015. If you recall from the introduction, there was a mention of oncoming symptoms. As the night took over the sky, the green highway signs started to look a little strange – like the writing was jumbled. The vision symptoms were sporadic. I was able to focus, but this was something new. As a distraction, I entertained my children by allowing them to DJ the music for the ride back. I engaged my son, Trey, with irrelevant conversation, which helped keep both of us alert. The other two slept the entire ride except for our frequent stops.

We made it back around 2:00 a.m. Monday morning. My vision seemed fine. I went to bed, awakened around 9:00 a.m. and prepared for work. Being an IT Professional for one of the biggest media companies in the world, my job is the resolve software and hardware issues. At the time, my shift was 12:30 p.m. through 9:00 p.m. I use three 17" monitors to complete my daily duties. I had a hard time focusing, having to squint in order to focus. On my ride home that night, the highway signs were doing that jumbling thing again and the red backlights of the cars in front of me looked like red triangles. I did not want to alert anyone, so I kept this to myself.

On Thursday, December 3, 2015, I received a voicemail from the doctor's office. The results were back from my labs. My A1c was 16.6.

What is A1c

A1c is a test that shows the average level of blood sugar over the past two-to-three months. Hemoglobin A1c (HgbA1c, HbA1c, or just A1c) is hemoglobin that has sugar attached to it. Hemoglobin is the protein that carries oxygen from the lungs to all the cells of the body. Once hemoglobin is glycated (covered with sugar), it stays that way until the red blood cell dies. Red blood cells live an average of three-to-four months. That is the reason why your A1c level indicates your average glucose over the last two-to-three months.

What is a Normal Range for A1c

There are several factors to consider when we discuss the normal range for A1c. I am only going to focus on normal for a Type 2 diabetic. Before eating or drinking anything in the morning, target blood sugar reading for non-pregnant adults with diabetes, otherwise known as fasting blood sugar and pre-meal blood sugar, is 80-130 mg/dl (milligrams per deciliter). Using a conversion calculator, an A1c of 5.1% would result in an average blood sugar reading of 100 mg/dl. Remember my A1c was 16.6%. Using a conversion calculator, my average blood sugar reading was 429 mg/dl. That is well over three times over normal. I could have had a stroke at any time.

That brings me back to our trip. Not only was I thirsty, but I was forgetful. I was not able to sing along with some of the songs. I was slurring some of the words and forgetting the lyrics. I would have conversations and forget what I had just spoke about or stop in mid-sentence. I actually showed early signs of a stroke and did not realize it. I also began to sort of walk with a limp. I felt like the arch of my foot was sore, so I just walked on the side of one foot. There were many signs. I am very grateful of the thirst problem that made me panic.

My doctor was able to get me in the next day, which was December 4, 2015. When the nurse took my blood sugar, it was 246. Still way too high. My doctor immediately put me on three different mediations and provided me with my very own Blood Glucose Monitoring Device. I began taking medication and monitoring my blood sugar numbers that same day.

My vision seemed to get worse even though I was on medication. I had a very hard time focusing. I remember waking up on that first Saturday, which was December 5th. I looked at my mobile phone to check the time and the light hurt my eyes; I was also unable to focus very well.

I tried to blink into focus to no avail. I was unable to read the numbers on my debit card. I was also unable to read the information on a can of soup or one of the scratch off lottery tickets I purchased on our ride back from Missouri. My eyes felt weird, like there was something in them.

High levels of blood sugar can cause fluid to leak into the lens of the eye making it swell and change shape. Glasses cannot correct this problem. Remember, I explained I was attempting to 'blink' into focus. At times, I was able to blink enough to see. However, my vision was still blurry.

I was instructed that weight loss and diet were very critical to getting my numbers down. My diet had to change. No more french fries, potato chips, grits, home fried potatoes, Big Macs, or watermelon chunks...Yes, watermelon chunks. At the time, I weighed 236 pounds. I have never been overweight even after having three children. I have never weighed over 165 pounds even during my pregnancies. I cannot explain the reason of the weight gain between the years 2010 and 2015. I can, however, explain how I took back my health. I learned the importance of watching carbs. I did not understand that carbohydrates turn into sugar. I have an older sister, who has been a nurse for over 40 years, who was very instrumental with my recovery.

I began my new diet Saturday, December 5, 2015. I went to the grocery store and purchased tomatoes, cucumbers, onions, Italian dressing, broccoli florets, and frozen fajita chicken and beef. For breakfast and lunch, I ate cucumber and tomato salad; for dinner, broccoli boiled with plant-based butter and the fajita chicken or beef.

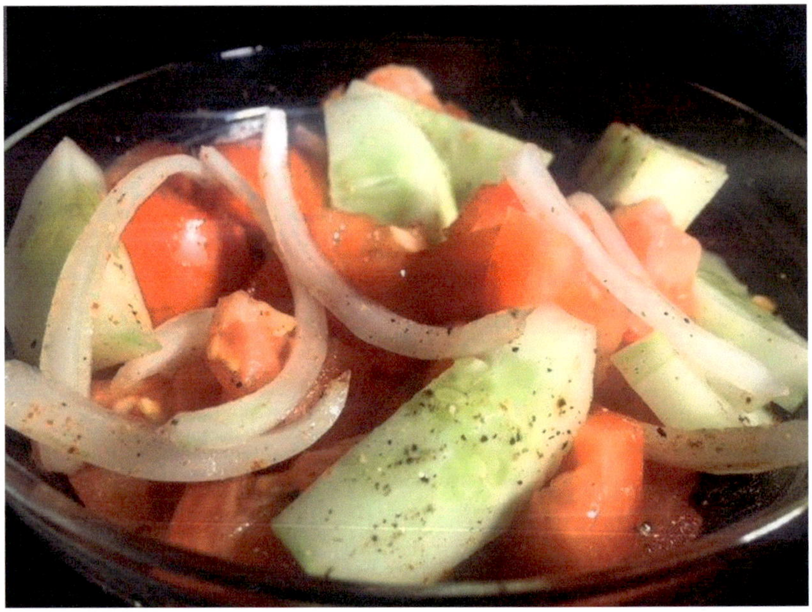

This was my meal consistently for the entire month of December. Other than drinking one glass of 2% milk per day, drank nothing but water. Since my blood sugar was so high, my doctor visits were set to every three weeks. By the time of my next scheduled appointment, I had lost almost 10 pounds. My weight went from 236 to 227. I still had the issue of blurred vision, but my eyes were not as sensitive to light. Each scheduled appointment showed a steady loss of weight. By the end of January, my size 18 clothes were loose. I was down to a size 16.

I began to add other items to my diet. I found cauliflower is a wonder vegetable. I created a dish for breakfast. I love home fried potatoes with onions and cheese. I chopped up a head of cauliflower, sliced some Vidalia onions, mixed the two, and added seasoning. Added extra virgin olive oil to the pan, fried my cauliflower and onions, and once nice and browned, added one slice of cheese. This dish was delicious. A coworker of mine asked me to bring her some the next day. She loved it.

This publication is not meant to be a 'How To' instructional. I want people to know my story and know healthy eating is delicious too. Being aware of what we eat and our family history can prevent such diseases like diabetes. Exercise is only a small piece of loving our bodies. Diet is the most important. Before changing my diet, exercise had no effect on my waistline. As of February 2018, I weighed 139 pounds and wear a size 4. No surgery. Just diet and exercise. My A1c at last check up was 5.8%.

Since I do have Type 2 diabetes, there are foods I exclude from my diet entirely:

- Pasta
- Bread
- Rice
- White Potatoes

I know, I know. I may as well starve. The four mentioned are foods easily found and require little to no preparation. They are the main ingredients in dishes at every restaurant and fast food places allowing us a quick, and in some cases, cheap meal. I learned how to substitute. I learned eating healthy is not always more expensive, you just make more trips to the store.

Pancreatic Function

Even if you do not have a family history of diabetes, watching your carb intake is still very important. The pancreas has a very important role. It produces enzymes and hormones that help you digest food. The pancreas produces insulin, which is one of the main hormones that helps to regulate blood glucose levels. The more sugars you put in your body, the harder the pancreas has to work. Over time, this can lead to insulin resistance. The result could lead to diabetes. If your pancreas stops producing the needed insulin, the result could also lead to having to give yourself insulin shots. I don't know about you, but I do not like needles.

Body Restoration

Diet is the key to restoring your body's health. Changing your diet is definitely more cost effective than tacking on doctors' bills and prescriptions. You would be surprised how eating well changes your mind, body, and spirit. It is also delicious. There are some combinations of vegetables I have never thought to try until I had to learn how to cook and eat differently. Again, this is not a book of instructions and lectures. I am not a dietician, nor am I a chef. I am a divorced mother of three who almost said an early goodbye to her children at the age of 42 due to ignoring my health.

When I cook and prepare my meals, I use simple, everyday ingredients. The only down side to eating healthy is you end up making more trips to the store. You cannot buy fresh fruit and vegetables in bulk. My recipes use simple spices like white salt, black pepper, garlic powder, Cajun seasonings, ginger, and zesty herb seasonings. I use a brand of butter that is plant-based, olive oil, and vegetable oil. Simple. I work the overnight shift, so I prepare my meals before going to sleep. My meals are usually something that I can throw together and have enough to last during my shift.

I hope you enjoy the simple recipe ideas I have put together to share with you…

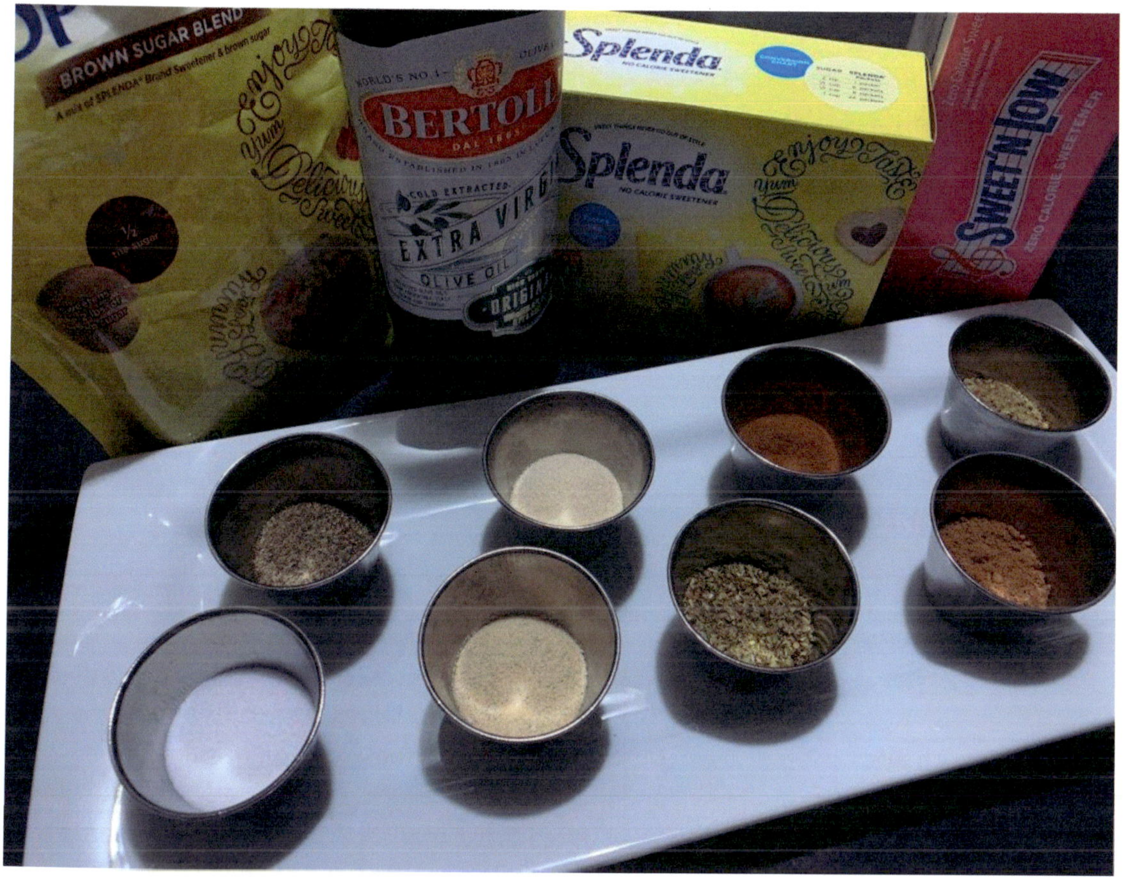
BROWN SUGAR BLEND
BERTOLLI
COLD EXTRACTED
OLIVE OIL
Splenda
NO CALORIE SWEETENER
Splenda
NO CALORIE SWEETENER
SWEET'N LOW
ZERO CALORIE SWEETENER

The Great Substitution

The following pages are recipes that I have compiled from experimenting and finding online. I have added my own touch to most. This is not a cookbook. I have learned how to substitute foods high in carbs with those of lower carb content. Therefore, the unhealthy, high carb foods are barely missed. Below, I have compiled a short list of those substitutes:

POPULAR CARB ITEM	SUBSTITUTE
Rice	Riced Cauliflower
Mashed Potatoes	Mashed Cauliflower
White Potatoes	Sweet Potatoes
Tortilla Chips	Bean Chips
Potato Chips	Sweet Potato Chips or Apple Chips
Spaghetti Pasta	Spaghetti Squash
Pasta	Spiraled Vegetables (Zucchini, Butternut Squash, etc.)
French Fries	Sweet Potato Fries
Bread	Lettuce
Pizza Crust	Pizza Crust made w/Cauliflower. The same recipe can be used to make a bun.

Fresh

Ground Ginger/Lemon/Mint/Cucumber

Drink

I used the internet to research home remedies for high blood sugar. I happened upon this delightful drink. Fresh ginger is a wonderful spice. It is loaded with nutrients that have powerful benefits for your body. The ability to lower your fasting A1c is one of those benefits. Usually, I prepare a cup of this refresher nightly for consumption or in the morning before I go to the gym.

- fresh ginger root
- lemon
- fresh mint leaves
- cucumber (1-2 slices)
- grater
- water

Grate ½ to 1 teaspoon of fresh ginger and add to a coffee cup of water. Cut lemon in half and squeeze one half of the lemon into your water. Add 2-3 mint leaves and 1-2 slices of cucumber.

Cover and place in the fridge overnight.

Drink this hot or cold. You can also add honey to sweeten or zero-calorie sweetener. I did not add the sweetener due to my high blood sugar.

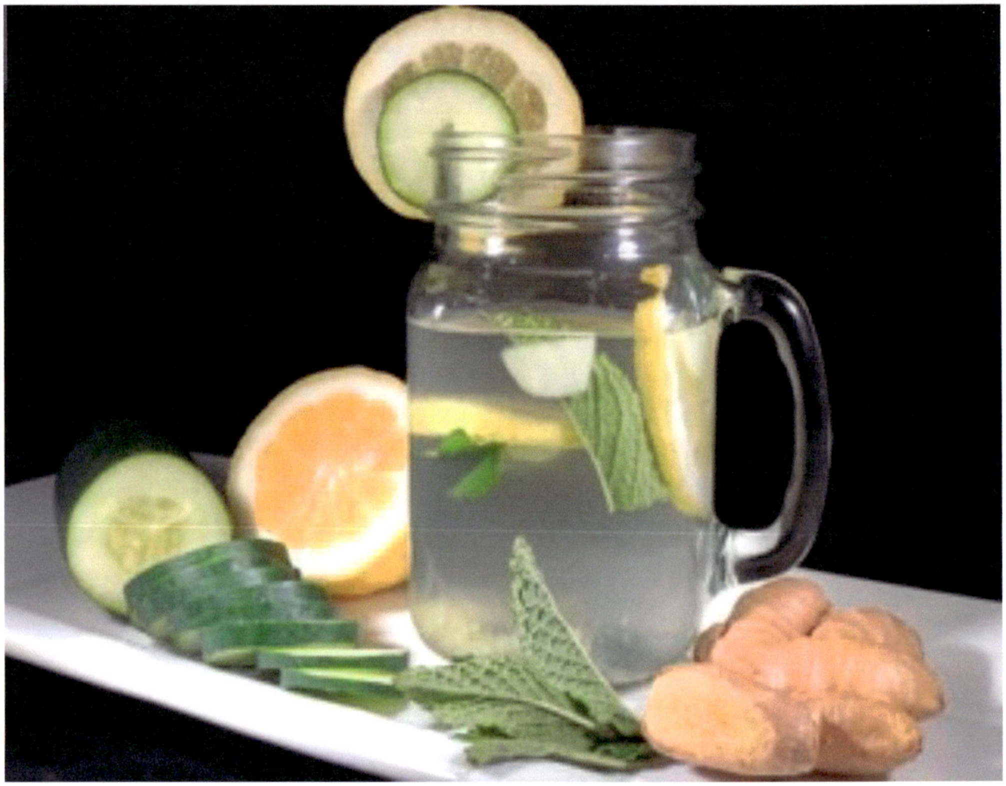

Sweet points for Kelli...

- Assisted with lowering my blood sugar
- Reduced my stomach bulge

I can be a witness to the results I received from consuming this drink daily before my workouts. Remember, I went from a size 20 to a 16 in less than 2 months. Yes, I really was a size 20. I refused to buy clothes that big!

Cauliflower Fried Rice

Fried rice is one of the dishes I really missed. I used to buy a container of beef fried rice every Saturday night to eat at my part-time job. I was crushed when I had to eliminate rice from my diet. I found this gem of a recipe on Pinterest. I have modified it with my personal touch. You would be amazed how great this dish mimics fried rice, minus the carbs.

- 1 (10 ounce) bag of riced cauliflower (you can rice it yourself or buy the frozen version with peas and carrots at your local grocery store)
- olive oil
- ¼ teaspoon white salt
- ¼ teaspoon black pepper
- 1 cup of Vidalia onions sliced or diced
- 1 cup of baby bella mushrooms
- ½ teaspoon garlic powder
- 1 cup chopped green onion
- cheesecloth or clean dish towel
- 1 cup of meat of your choice
- 2 tablespoons soy sauce (reduced sodium version – more can be used if preferred)
- 1 egg fried (optional)

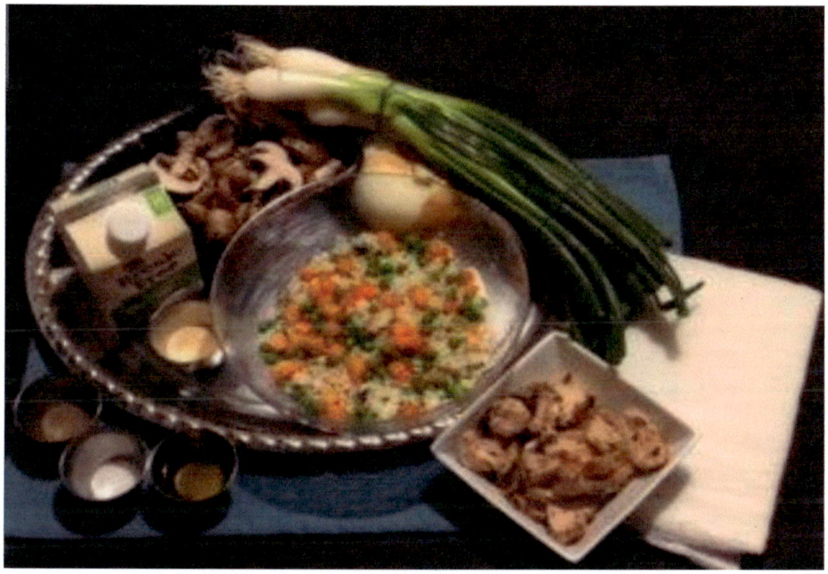

For the sake of simplicity, I use the version of riced cauliflower found in the frozen vegetable section with peas and carrots.

First, place the bag of riced cauliflower in the microwave for about 3 minutes. If you are using more than one bag, you will need to microwave them one-by-one. Empty the contents of the bag(s) onto the cheesecloth or towel. Squeeze out all of the moisture (this is a very important step). Set to the side.

Dice or slice your Vidalia onion, baby bella mushrooms, and green onions.

Add olive oil to grease a heated pan. Add the diced/sliced Vidalia onions and mushrooms. Sauté until the onions are slightly caramelized. Add riced cauliflower. Season with salt, pepper, and garlic powder to taste. Stir-fry until you have a little color. Add your meat of choice along with green onion and soy sauce.

If you want to add the fried egg, use a separate pan to fry the egg and add to the meat, green onion, and soy sauce. If you are a creative cook, just make a hole in the middle of your cauliflower rice, add a little olive oil then crack the egg and let it fry.

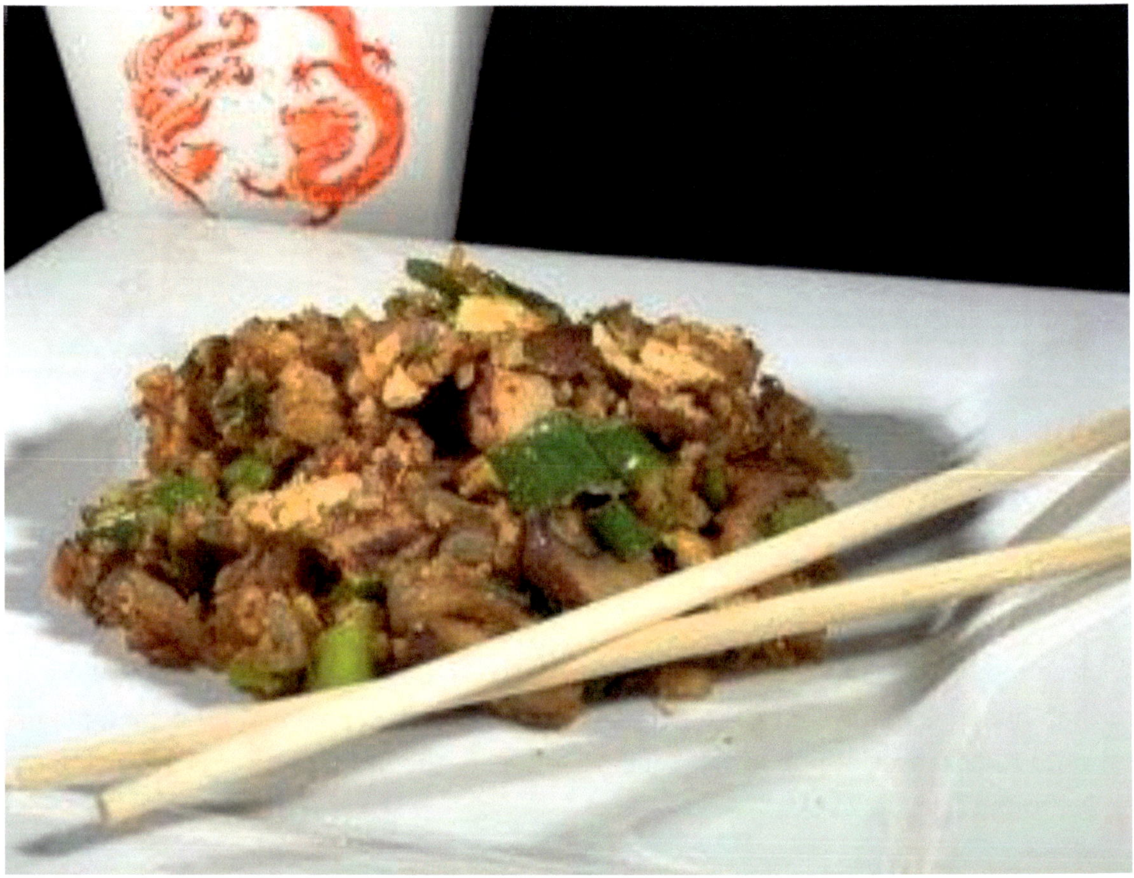

Nachos

How about some tasty nachos? The meat of choice is ground chicken and the chips of choice are bean chips. Remember, as a diabetic, simple substitutions are a must. Adding ground chicken is a preference. However, bean chips are the important substitute. The bean chip of choice has no flour or corn. Both flour and corn can cause your blood sugar to spike.

- 1 pound ground meat (chicken is pictured)
- 1½ packages of taco seasoning (brand package)
- 2 cups of lettuce diced (red leaf lettuce is pictured)
- ⅓ cup sweet onion
- ½ cup green diced green onions
- 3-4 diced tomatoes (Plum/Roma tomatoes pictured)

Chop lettuce, tomatoes, sweet onions, and green onions. Set all to the side except for the sweet onions.

Add the sweet onions and meat to pan. Since we are using ground chicken, we will add a little olive oil to the pan also. Brown your meat and onions. No need to drain. Add taco seasoning and water according to directions on the package. Let simmer until most of the water has cooked down.

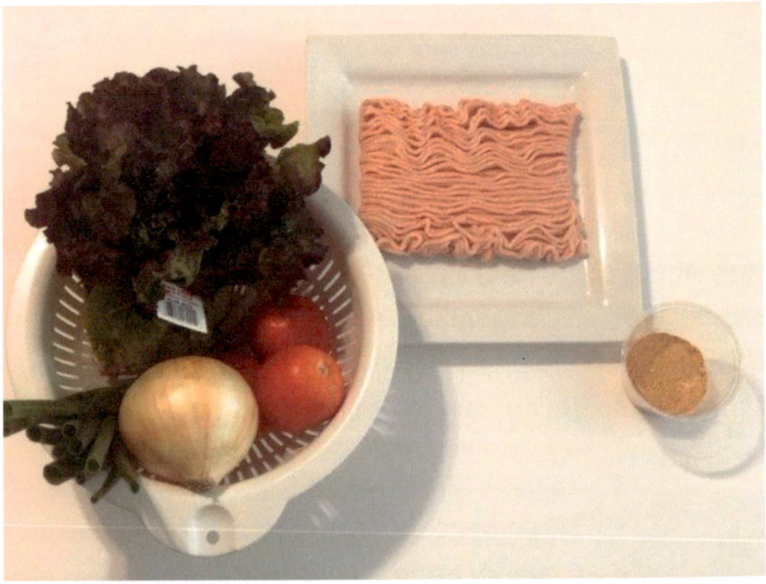

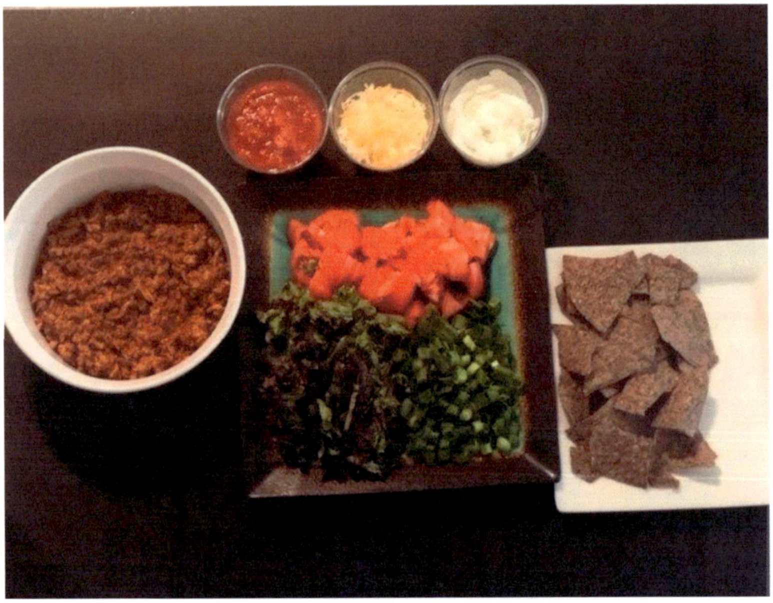

To complete your nachos, break out the following items:

- chunky salsa
- shredded cheese (Mexican mix pictured)
- sour cream
- bean chips

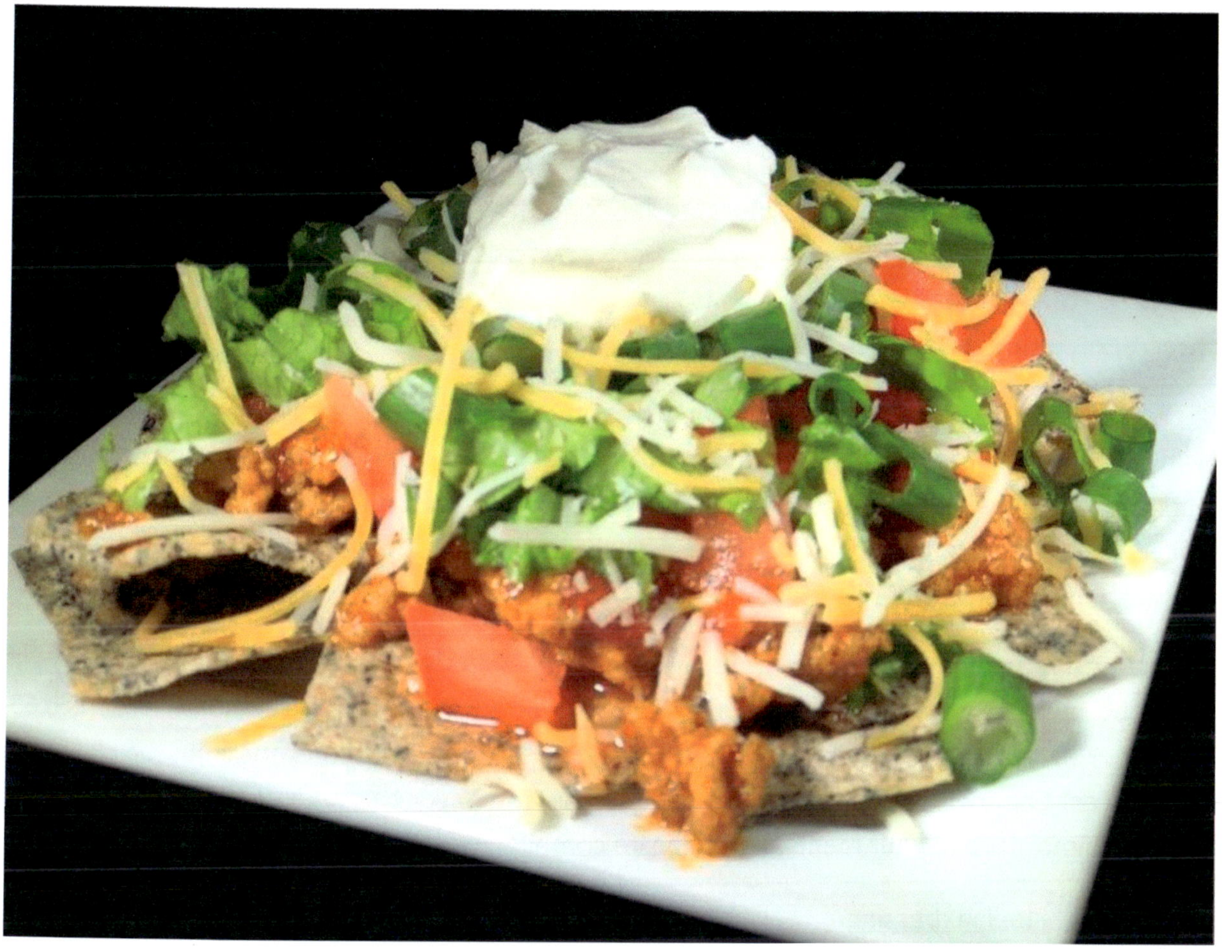

Grilled Chicken

One of the best skills I have learned in recent years is how to use a grill. Fried foods are a diabetic's enemy due to the high saturated fat content and the breading. I love baked foods, but the taste of grilled meats and vegetables are a symphony to my pallet. A great way to save money is to have tasty cooked meats and vegetables pre-cooked and ready for quick preparation by grilling and freezing them.

Of course, the headliner is the seasonings. Remember, I use simple everyday seasonings for all of my foods. I am not a chef. The rock star of my grilled meats is zesty herb seasonings and marinades. You can make your own or buy them already bottled or packaged at your local grocer. In the picture below, I have used a packaged version of zesty herb seasoning on my skinless boneless chicken breasts.

To ensure the best outcome, I do not place my meats directly over the heat. This process will allow the meat to slow cook and smoke. The safe internal temp for cooked chicken is 165 degrees. You can add other flavoring agents to your coals such as hickory chips or chopped onions…Yes! Chopped onions! You would not believe the flavor this adds to grilled burgers. To ensure the moisture of your meats, I use a baste compiled with the following ingredients:

- Italian dressing
- Worcestershire sauce
- Teriyaki sauce
- soy sauce
- Liquid smoke

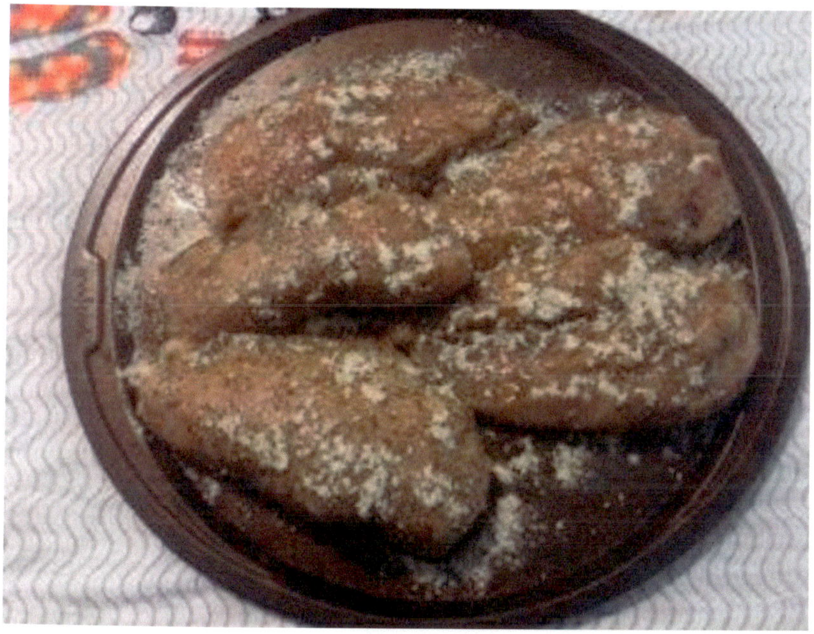

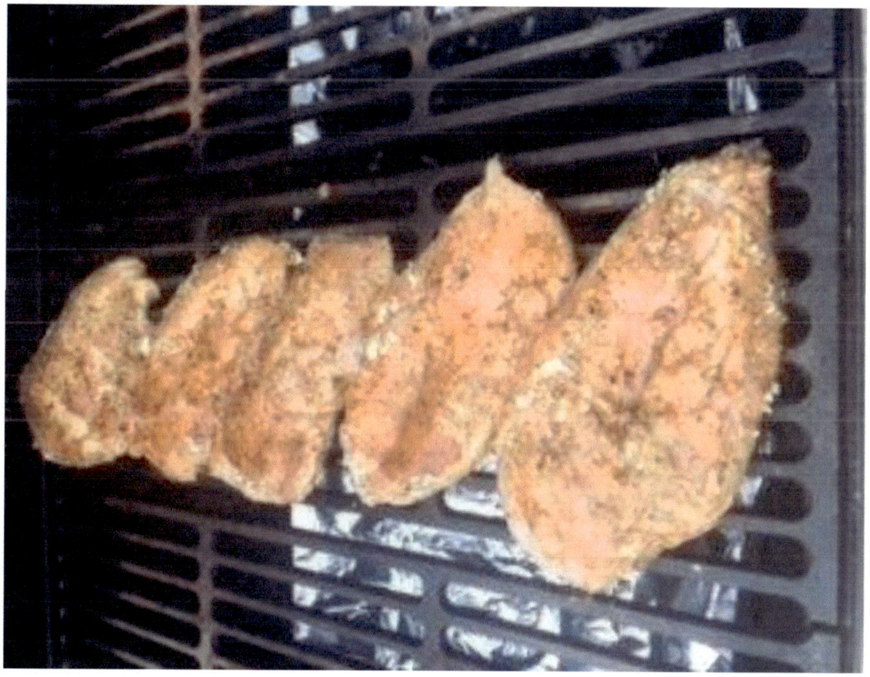

Grilled Brussel Sprouts/Mushrooms/Onions

This dish I usually sauté; however, grilling took the flavor from delicious to off of the charts!

Ingredients:

- Brussel sprouts (6-10 halved and chopped to look liked sliced cabbage)
- sliced baby portabella mushrooms
- sliced onions
- white salt
- black pepper
- garlic powder
- extra virgin olive oil
- soy sauce

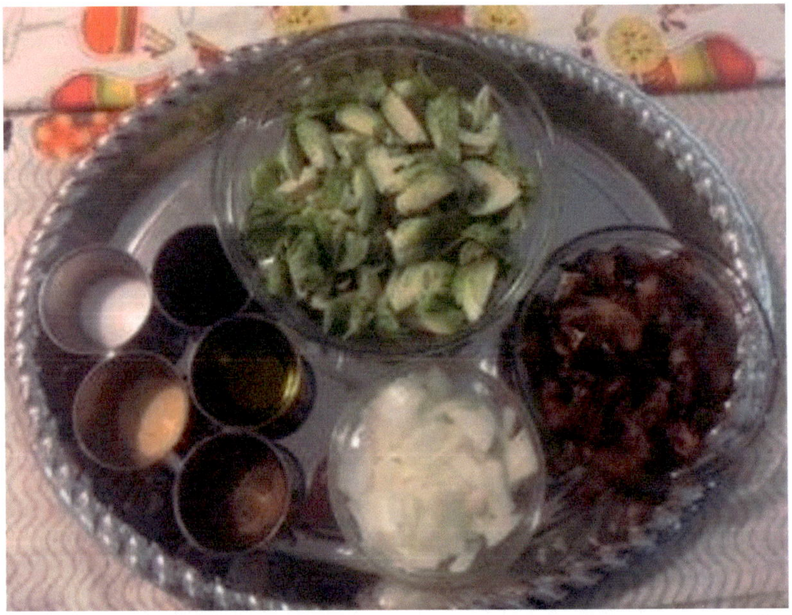

Place all of your vegetables in a large bowl. Add dry seasoning. I do not use measure-ments, season to taste. Toss in about 3 tablespoons of extra virgin olive oil.

Place vegetables in a pan made to use on the grill. Grill until tender. Add soy sauce right before removing from the grill.

The result is a bowl full of grilled vegetable deliciousness...

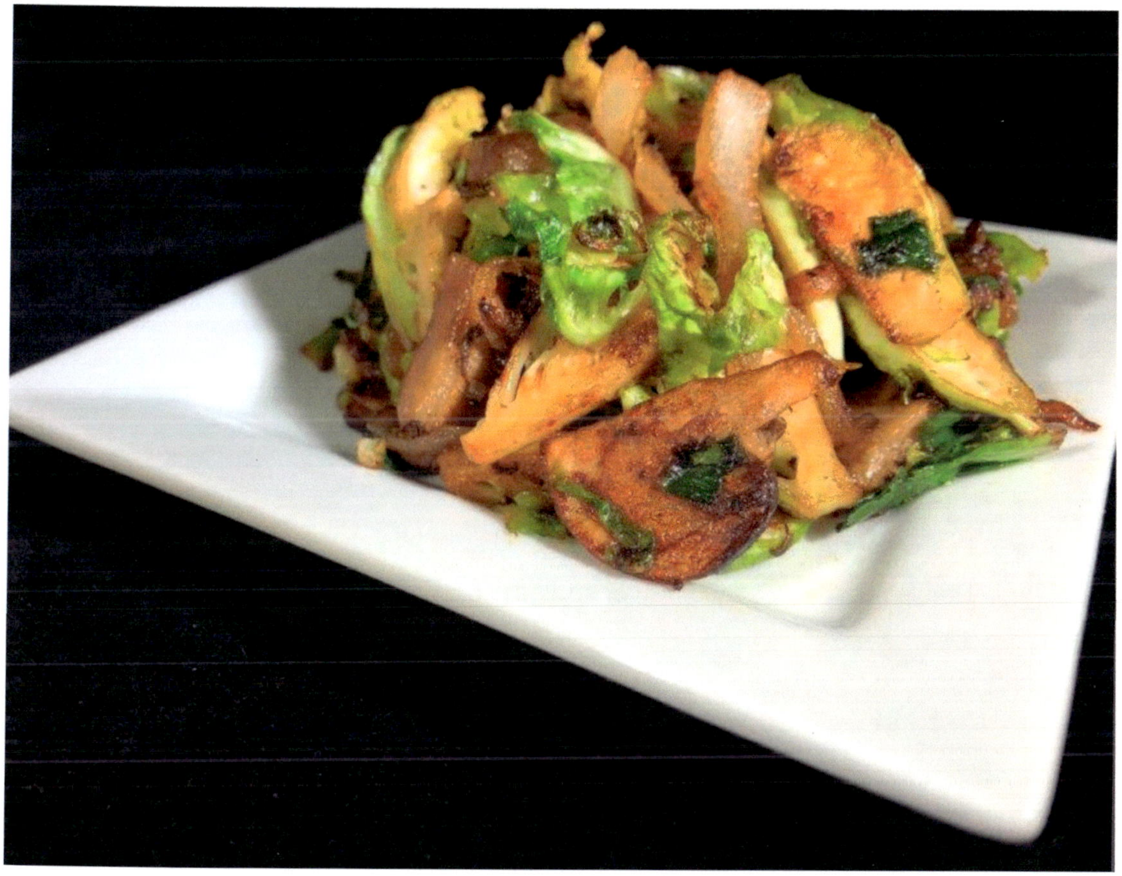

Eggroll In A Bowl

I love eggrolls. There are around 16-20 carbs in the wrappers. To eliminate that, I've found a tasty substitute simply called 'Eggroll in a bowl.' It's the eggroll without the wrapper! You will need the following ingredients:

- 1 (16 ounce) roll of ground sausage (I used chicken, but Jimmy Dean has Cajun seasoned sausage that is perfect for this dish. Slice the sausage in half, use your fingers to get the meat out of the casing. Use all four sausages that come in the package.)
- 1 (16 ounce) bag of coleslaw mix
- ½ cup sliced Vidalia onion
- ¼ cup green onions chopped
- ¼ teaspoon black pepper
- ¼ teaspoon garlic powder
- 1 tablespoon extra virgin olive oil
- 1 tablespoon soy sauce (lower sodium content)

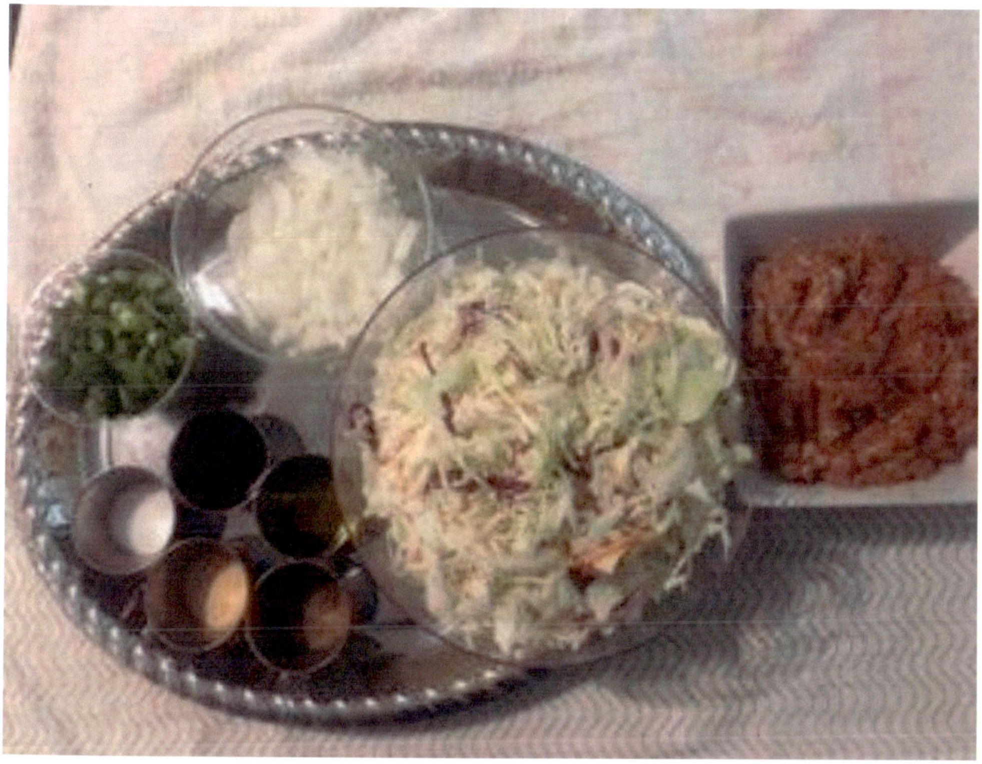

Since the chicken sausage does not have the fat content of pork sausage, add about a tablespoon of extra virgin olive oil to your pan. Brown your sausage along with the sliced onion.

Once the sausage has browned, add the cabbage mix. Add pepper and garlic powder. Please watch your seasonings. I excluded salt on purpose. Adding salt can make this dish too salty.

Once the cabbage has cooked down, add the green onions and about a tablespoon of soy saucc.

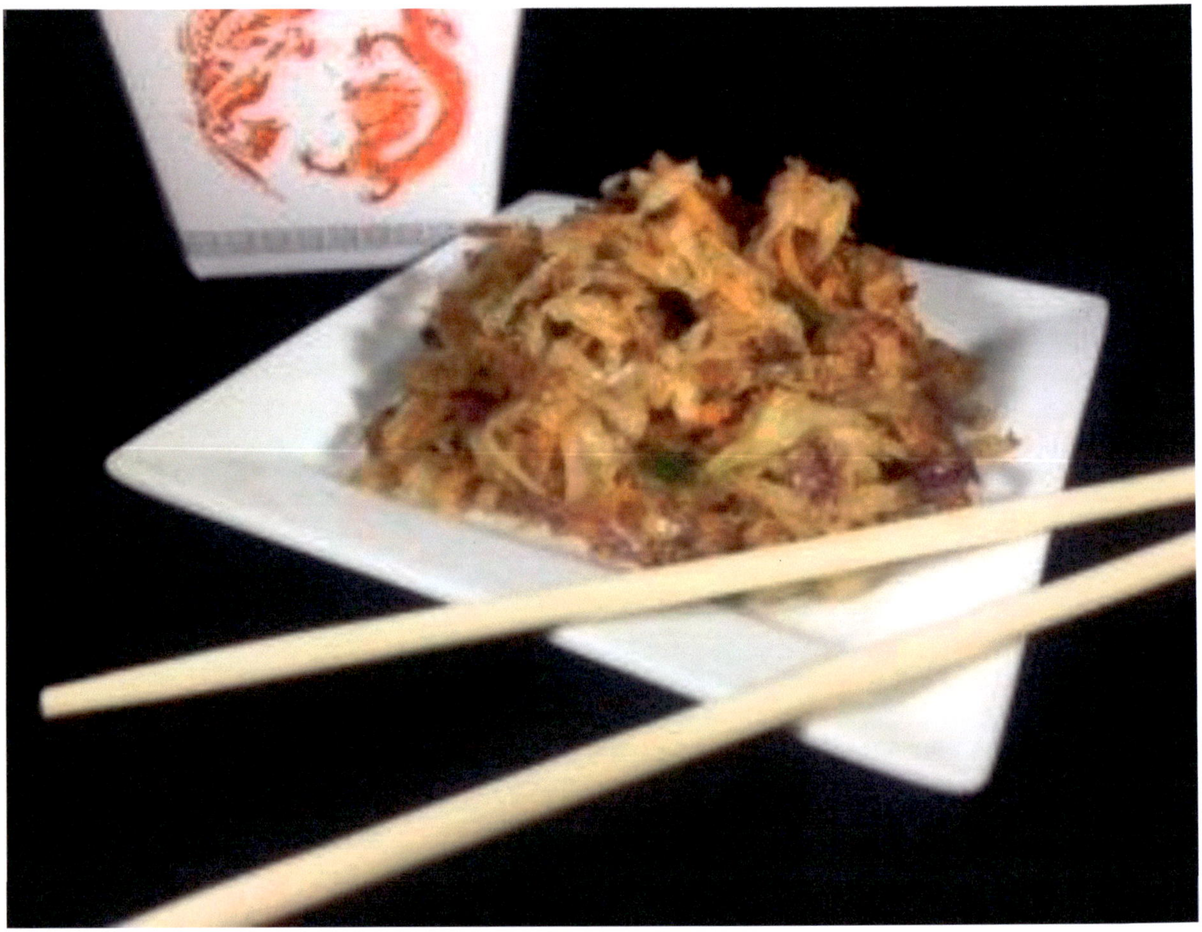

Food For Thought NUMBer 1...

While in the process of creating this book, my sister reminded me about my 'fasting' readings versus the readings after having something to eat and/or drink. When my initial A1c readings came back, my Fasting A1c was 16.6% which averaged 429. Imagine what it must have been after consuming a meal... The thought is extremely frightening. I know my pancreas was having all sorts of temper tantrums!

Stuffed Avocado

The avocado is rich in vitamins and minerals. They are a great source of vitamins C, E, K, and B-6. They are also a source of riboflavin, niacin, folate pantothenic acid, magnesium, and potassium. This small giant supports skin health, heart health, vision, and is a natural detox source. Avocados contain healthy fat. Eating fat slows the breakdown of carbs, which in return helps to keep sugar levels in the blood stable.

I remember my first taste of guacamole. I had no idea what this green stuff was. I was at a hotel with an up and coming R&B artist, guacamole with pretzel sticks was one of the appetizers. I had to ask one of the staff members what was I eating. He advised me it was guacamole, which is made from avocados. Since that day, I never made tacos or nachos without having guacamole on the side.

This stuffed avocado recipe can be used with a variety of ingredients. I used the following:

- ½ cup of cooked chicken (I used the meat from three drumsticks that have been skinned, seasoned, and baked. You can also use canned meat.)
- ¼ cup of sundried tomatoes (chopped small)
- ¼ cup green onion (chopped)
- ¼ teaspoon of white salt
- ¼ teaspoon of black pepper
- 1 teaspoon of lime juice

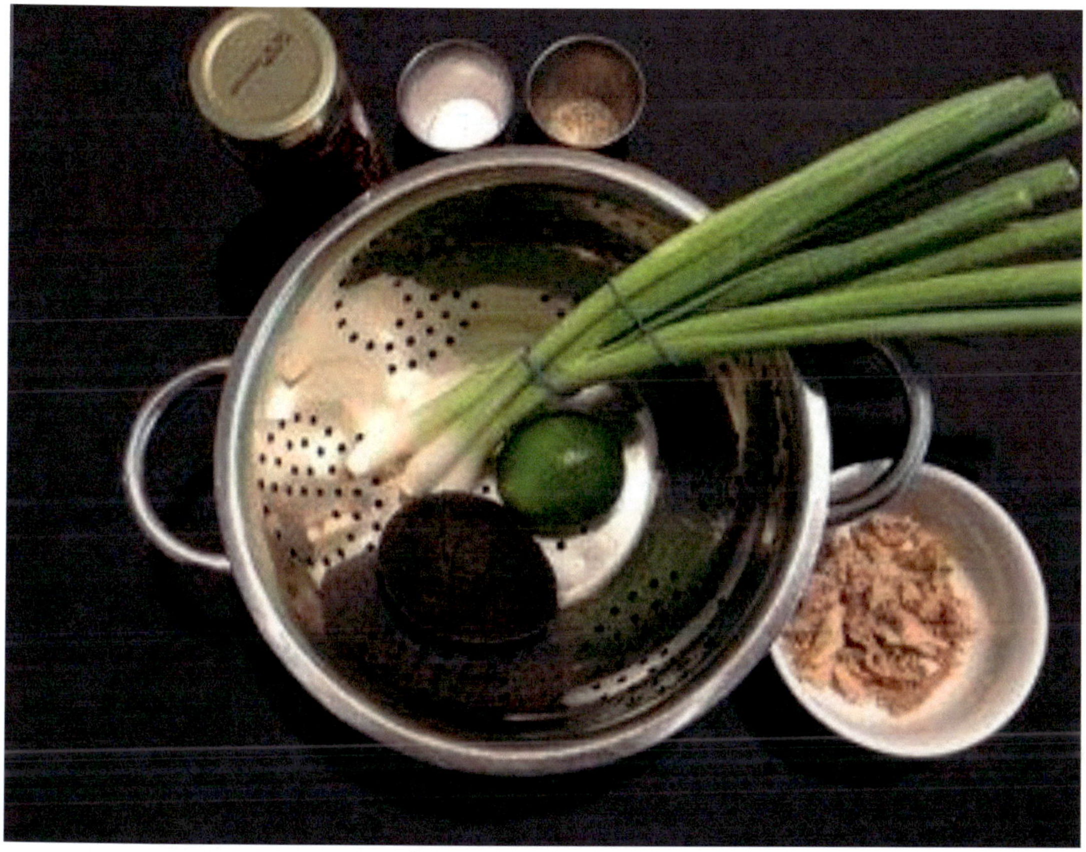

Half the avocado and remove the seed. Use a spoon to scoop the meat of the avocado out of each half into a bowl. Add lime juice to keep the avocado meat from browning. Do not throw away the shell. Mash the meat of the avocado and add chicken, sundried tomatoes, green onions, salt and pepper.

Mix ingredients using a spoon. Add your mixture back to the shell halves. I promise your palate will sing with joy!

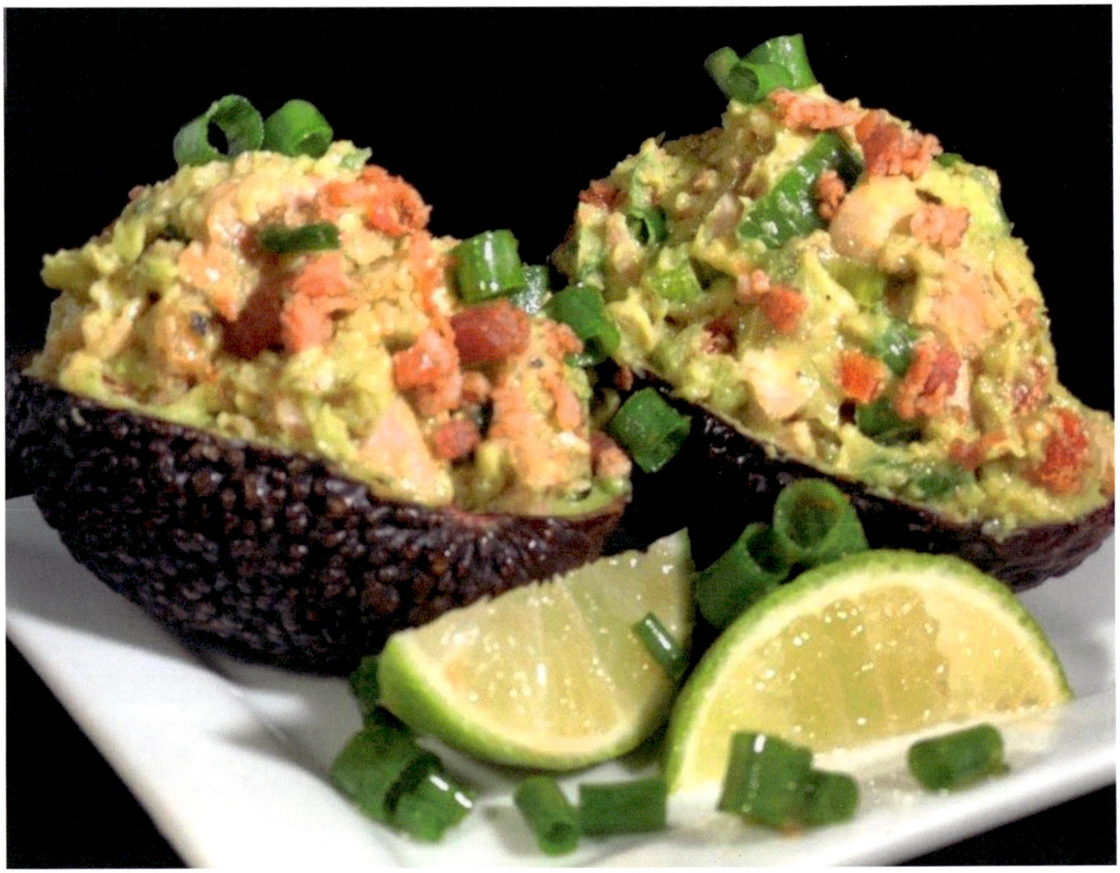

Cucumber and Tomato Salad

This dish was my savior! I prepared this dish religiously for the first 3 months of my diet change. I recall my sister bursting my bubble by telling me, "Tomatoes have carbs, Kelli." *Noooooooooo*! I still made this salad daily.

- 3-4 tomatoes sliced (I used Roma)
- 1 cucumber sliced
- Vidalia onion (⅛ sliced or chopped)
- ¼ teaspoon white salt
- ¼ teaspoon black pepper
- a dash of cayenne pepper
- Italian dressing

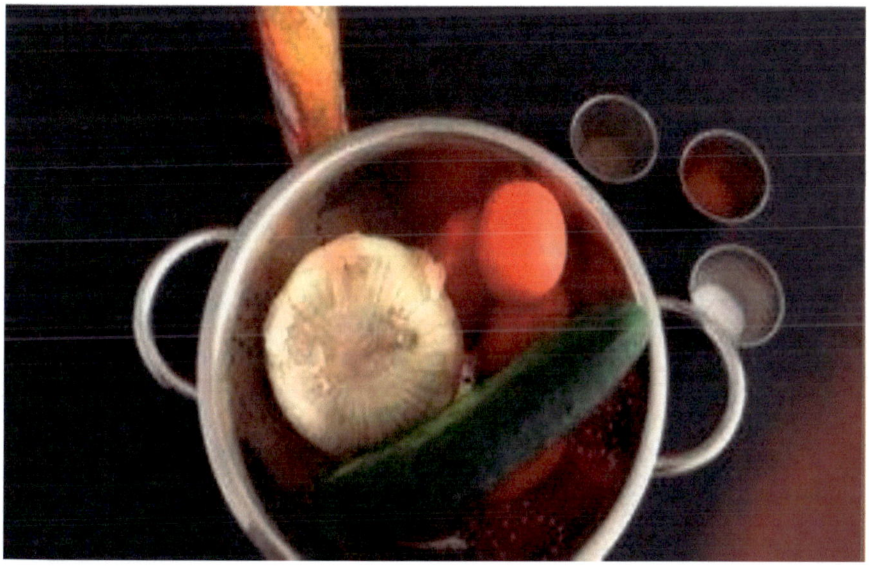

Slice your vegetables and add to a bowl. Season with a pinch of salt, black pepper, and cayenne pepper. Do not add the dressing to your ingredients bowl. It will become watered down and will lose the rich, tangy flavor.

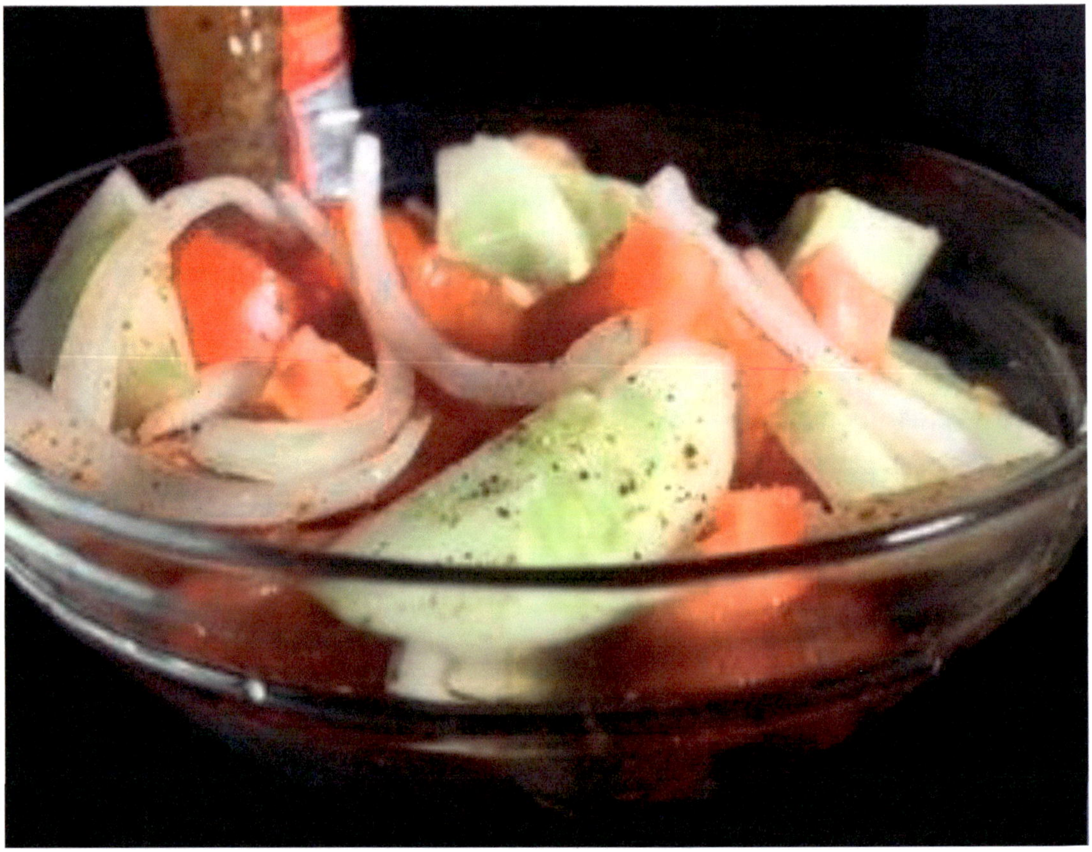

Zoodles, Meatballs, and Spaghetti Sauce

I love spaghetti. I have missed spaghetti. Pasta and rice are the enemy to a diabetic. Thank goodness for this great pasta substitute: spiraled zucchini noodles.

- spiraled zucchini noodles
- meatballs (pre-packaged were used)
- jar of favorite spaghetti sauce (making your own is even better)
- extra virgin olive oil

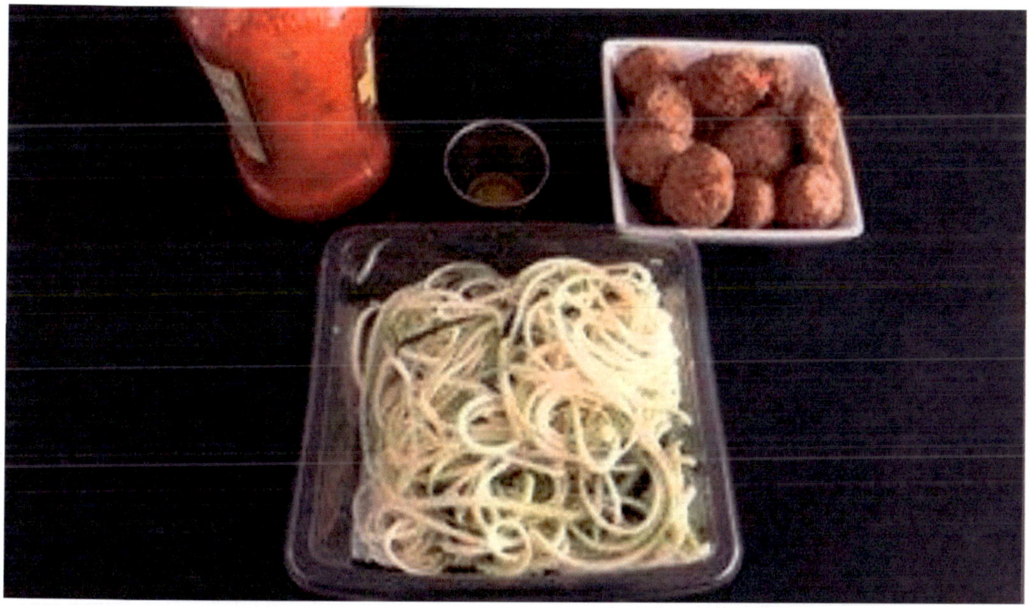

Add olive oil to pan and heat. Add zoodles to pan and sauté 3-5 minutes.

Add meatballs and spaghetti sauce. Cook until sauce and meatballs are thoroughly heated. You can also heat meatballs and sauce separately then add them to the pan.

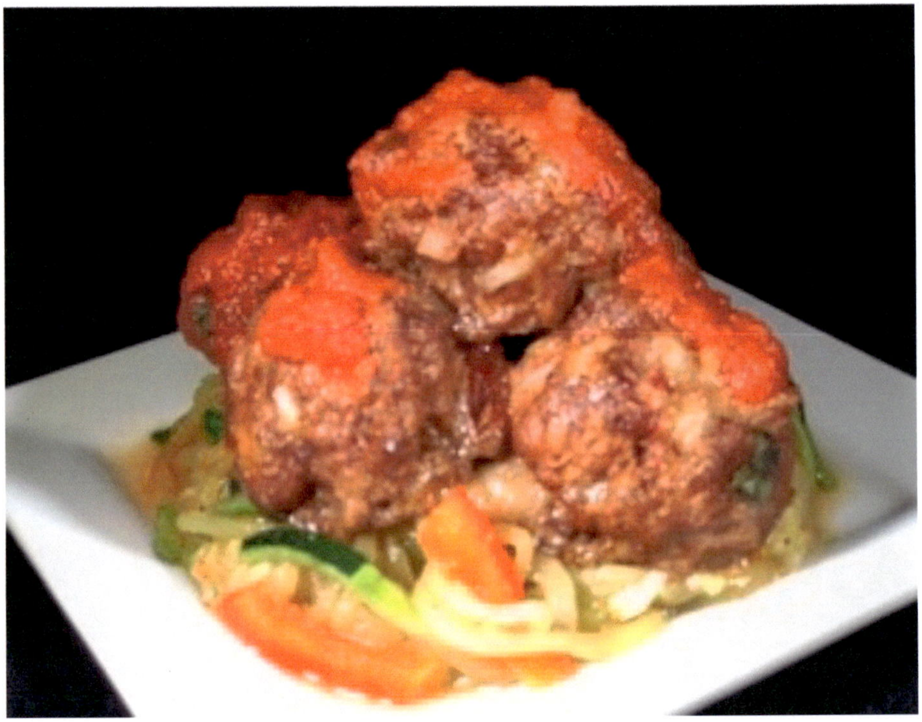

Homemade Meatballs

I wanted to elaborate on the previous recipe. Making your own meatballs or meat sauce is just as easy as using store bought. Since I do not eat pork, buying beef meatballs is next to impossible. Most are comprised of both beef and pork. Making your own meatballs is very easy. The benefit of course is knowing exactly what ingredients are being used.

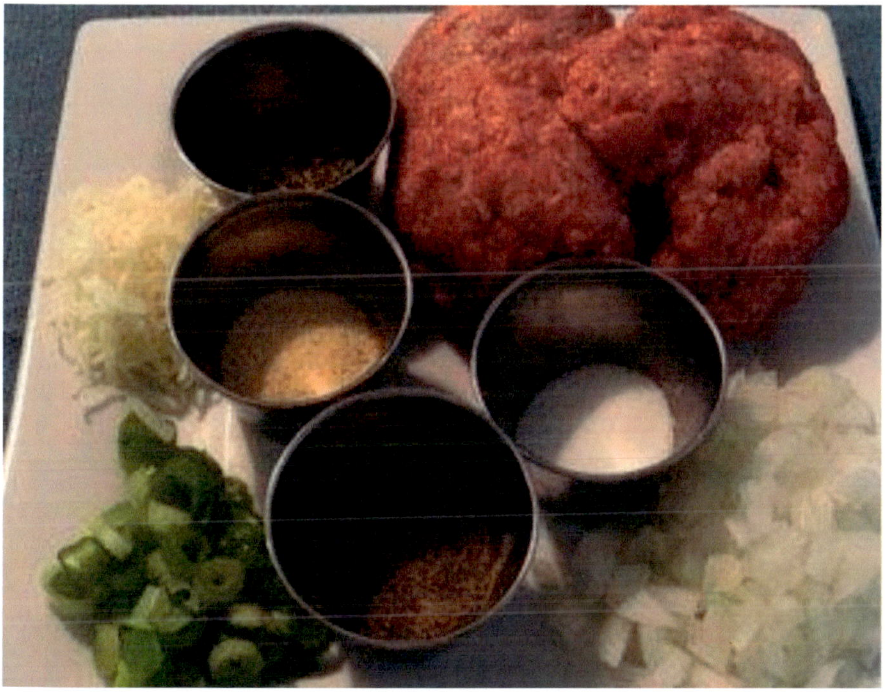

You will need the following:

- 1 pound ground meat (pictured is ground beef)

- ½ cup chopped onion (pictured is Vidalia)
- ¼ teaspoon white salt
- ¼ teaspoon black pepper
- ¼ teaspoon garlic powder
- ½ teaspoon ground oregano
- ½ cup of mozzarella cheese
- ¼ cup green onions chopped

Some of the above ingredients are optional. Since you are making this masterpiece, you can add a variety of seasonings.

Preheat oven to 350 degrees.

Place ground meat, onion (Vidalia and green), mozzarella cheese, and all of the spices in a bowl and mix. Some like to add egg to their meat as a binder.

Use an ice cream scooper or a teaspoon to evenly portion the mixture, then roll into a ball. Place meatballs into a baking pan. Bake for about 30 minutes or until fully cooked.

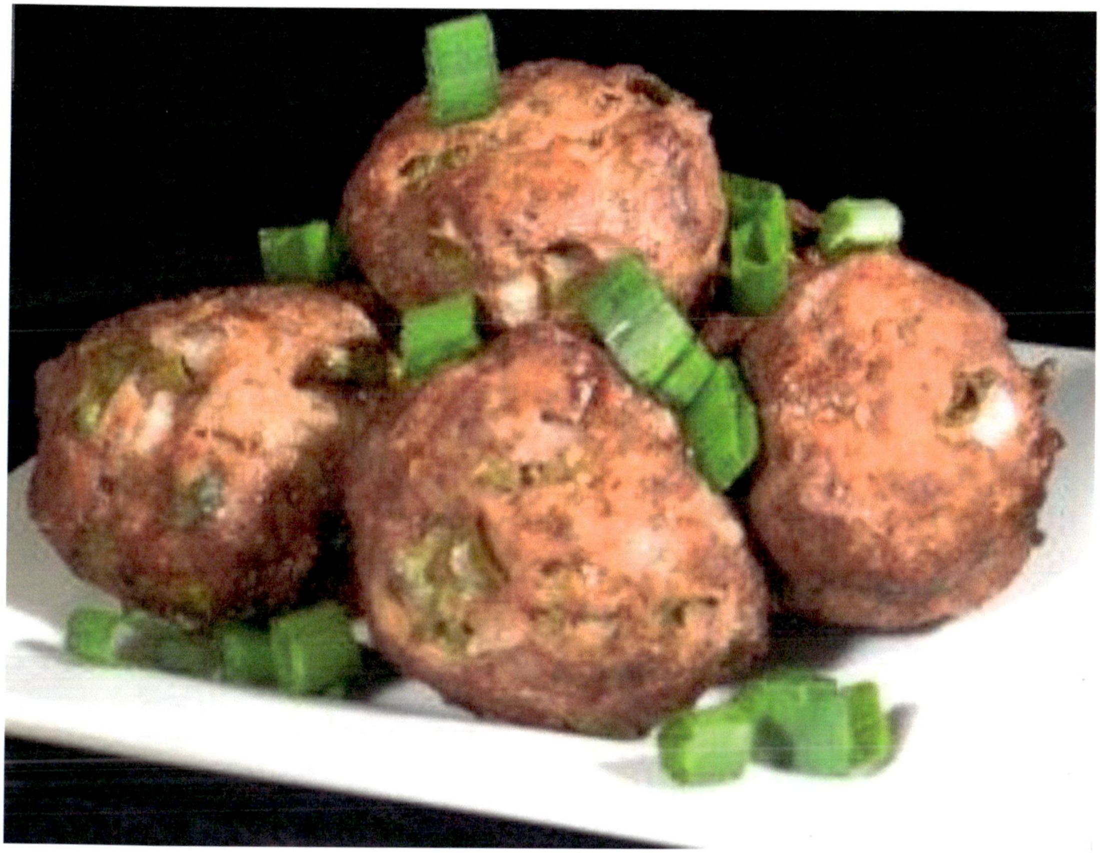

Split Pea Soup with Smoked Turkey

Split pea soup is one of my absolute favorite soups! I will tell you that even though this is a vegetable, peas can be a diabetic's enemy. Both peas and corn contain carbs, however the fiber and protein content of peas are thought to help slow digestion, which can help smooth out blood sugar levels after eating.

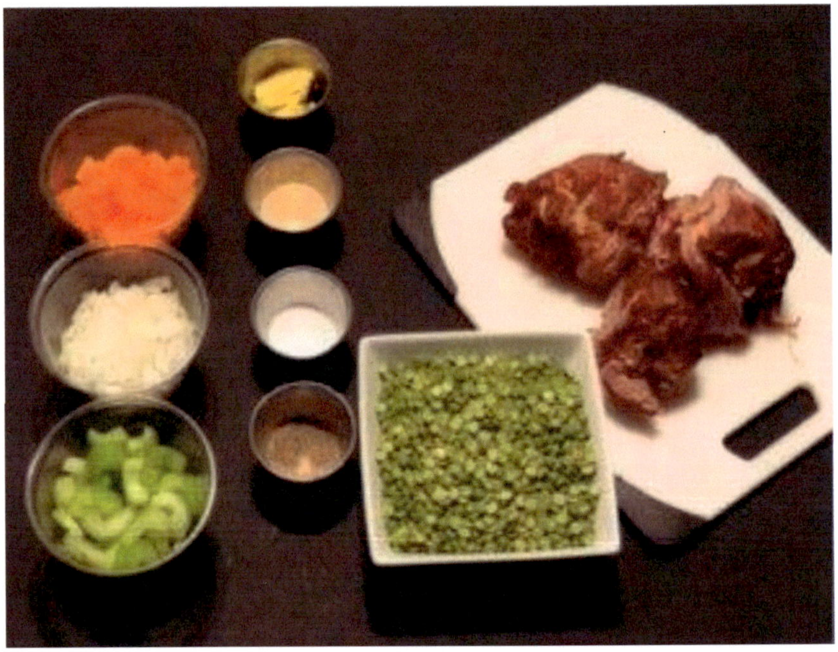

To create this wonderful green masterpiece, you will need the following:

- 1 (16 ounce) package of split peas
- smoked turkey (pictured are smoked turkey necks)
- 1 cup of chopped celery
- 1 cup of chopped carrots
- 1 cup of chopped onions
- ½ teaspoon white salt
- ½ teaspoon black pepper
- ½ teaspoon garlic powder
- 2 tablespoons chicken powder
- 2 cups chicken broth
- 4-5 cups of water

Place all of your ingredients in a crock pot. As far as measurements go with the spices, season to taste. The measurements provide a baseline.

Fill your crock pot with chicken broth and water. Make sure that the amount of liquid used covers your ingredients and is at least half of an inch past the top of your ingredients. Set your crock-pot to cook slow for 6 hours.

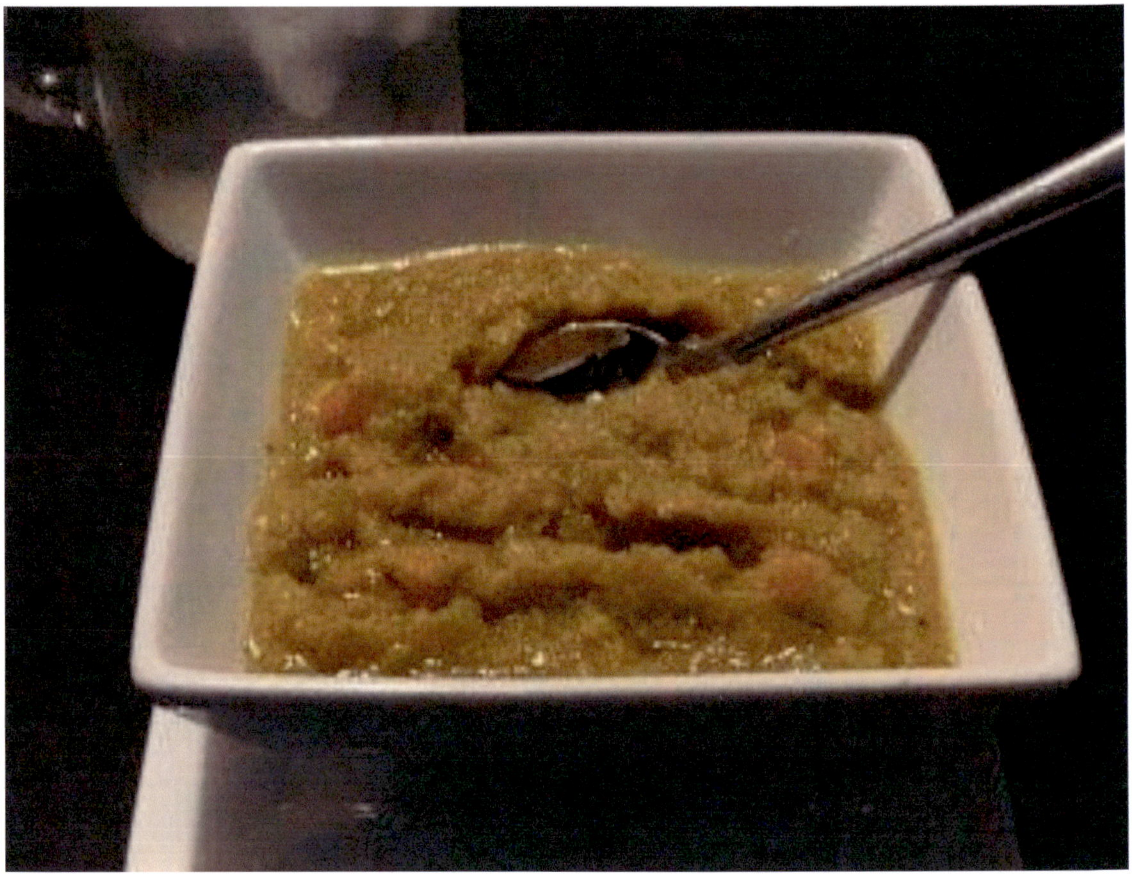

Sautéed Cabbage w/Grilled Chicken

I usually prepare this dish using grilled turkey legs. You can use whatever type of meat you would like. You can also make this a vegan dish by using mushrooms and a variety of other vegetables.

You will need the following:

- 1 head of green cabbage
- 1 Vidalia onion
- 1 red bell pepper
- 1 bunch of green onions
- white salt
- black pepper
- garlic powder
- chicken bouillon (1-2 cubes)
- meat of choice (Pictured is grilled chicken)

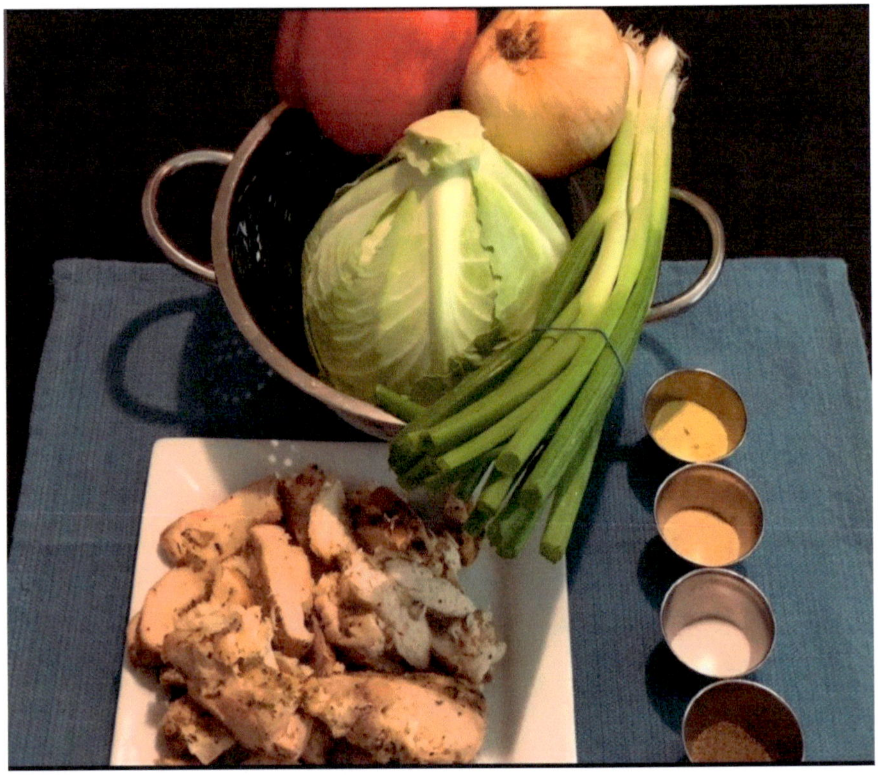

Chop cabbage into fine slivers; chop Vidalia onion, green onion, and bell pepper; chop green onions and set to the side.

Add olive oil to your pan on medium heat. Once your pan is hot enough, add your cabbage, Vidalia onion, bell pepper, and seasoning. Sauté until cabbage has cooked down to almost done. Add your meat and green onions and cook for another 3-4 minutes to incorporate the taste of your meat.

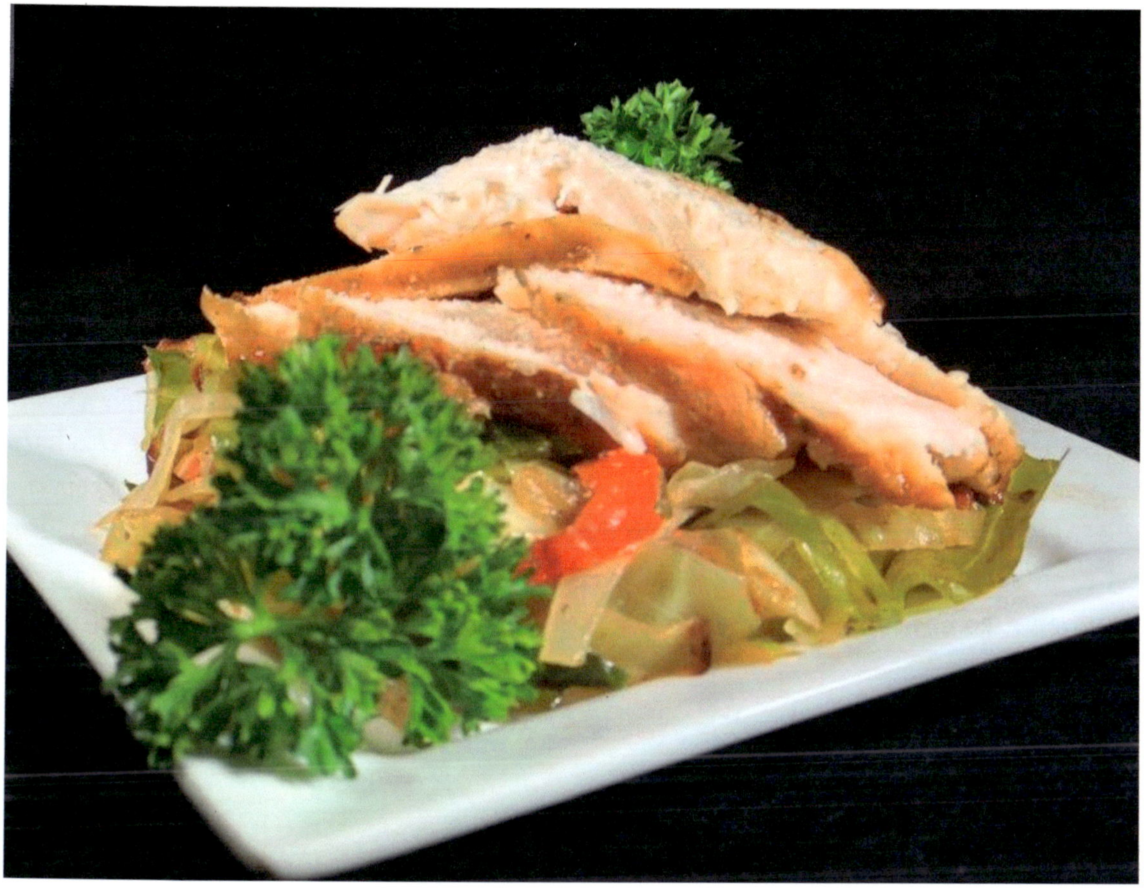

Red bell pepper adds so much color. You can also use orange and/or yellow bell peppers.

Food For Thought NUMBer 2...

A colleague and I took a challenge recently. We ate like vegans for 30 days. I actually extended my challenge to 60 days. Our diet consisted of fruit, vegetables, and nuts, though it was hard to give up meats and dairy products. I will say that after the first 5 days, I did not miss eating meat. My body felt different. My digestive system moved like, "Atlanta traffic on Christmas Day." My sweat even smelled different. It really had no smell! Do not be afraid to step outside of your norm when it comes to improving your diet. Most of my featured dishes can be easily made into vegan dishes.

Cauliflower Pizza Crust

One popular meal I really missed was pizza. My favorite includes extra cheese, hamburger, Canadian bacon, onions, and even more cheese. Have you taken a look at the carbs and sugars in the crust of your favorite pizza? You are looking at almost 40 grams per slice! That is #teamtoomuch!

So when I found this gem on the internet, I almost cried with joy.

Your ingredients will include:

- Riced cauliflower (you can rice yourself or buy the frozen version from your local grocery store. If you rice it yourself, use one head of cauliflower. One bag of riced cauliflower was used.)
- 1 egg
- ⅓ cup of grated Parmesan cheese
- ¼ cup of shredded mozzarella cheese
- ½ teaspoon of dried oregano
- ½ teaspoon of white salt
- ¼ teaspoon of garlic power
- ½ teaspoon of red pepper flakes
- cheesecloth or clean dish towel
- parchment paper

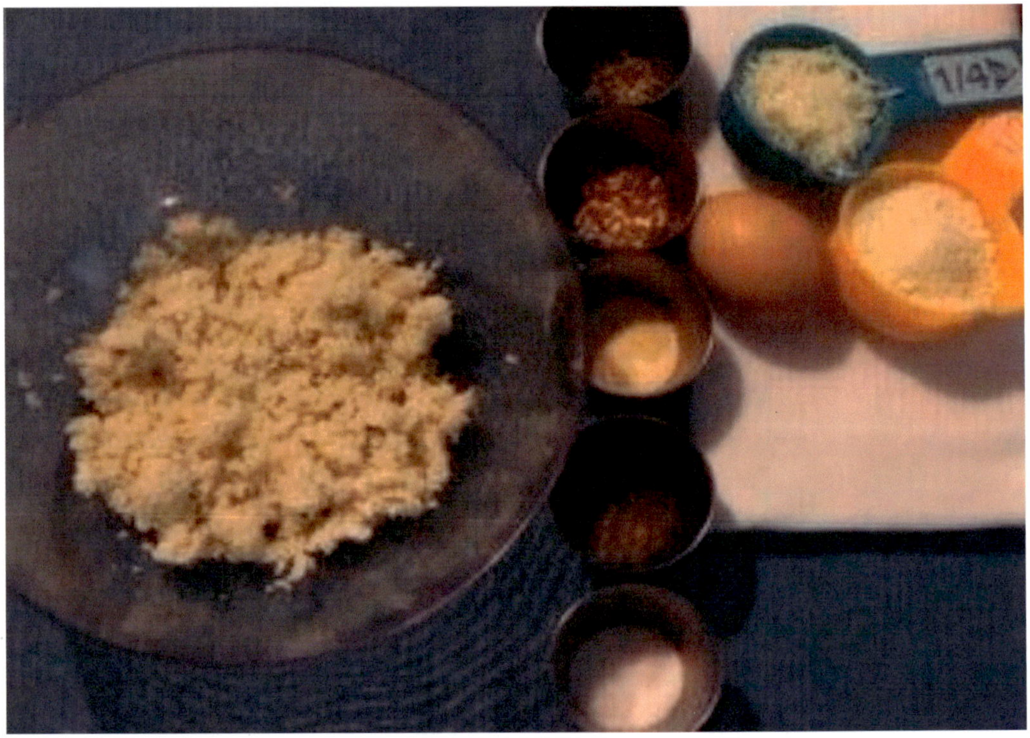

Preheat oven to 400 degrees.

If you rice the cauliflower, you will need to steam in a steamer basket for approximately 5-7 minutes. If you buy the frozen riced cauliflower, microwave it for 3-4 minutes to thaw. Use your cheesecloth or dishtowel to squeeze all of the moisture out. Very important. If you do not squeeze out the moisture, you will end up with a pile of mush. Set in a bowl.

Mix in your cheeses, spices, and egg; incorporate well. Line your cookie sheet with parchment paper. Shape your crust mixture.

Your finished product should look like the picture below:

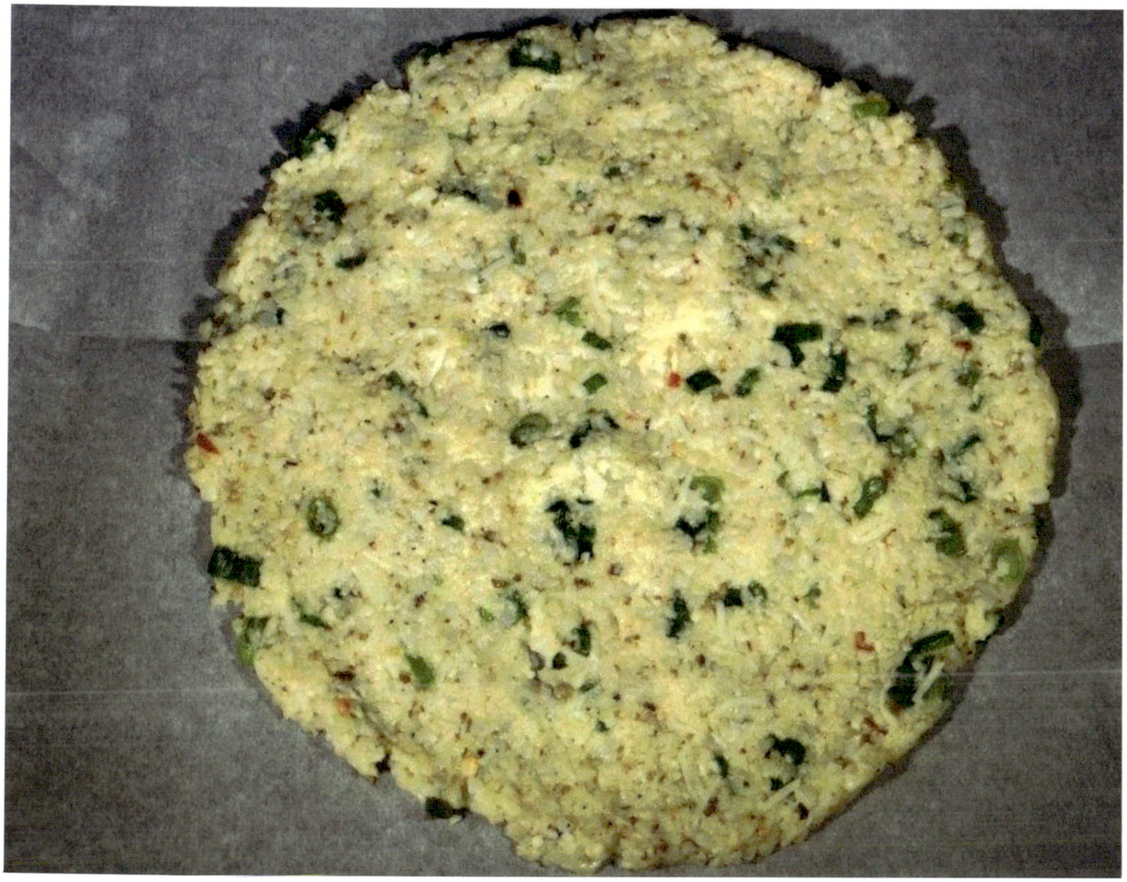

Bake your crust for around 30-40 minutes or until golden brown.

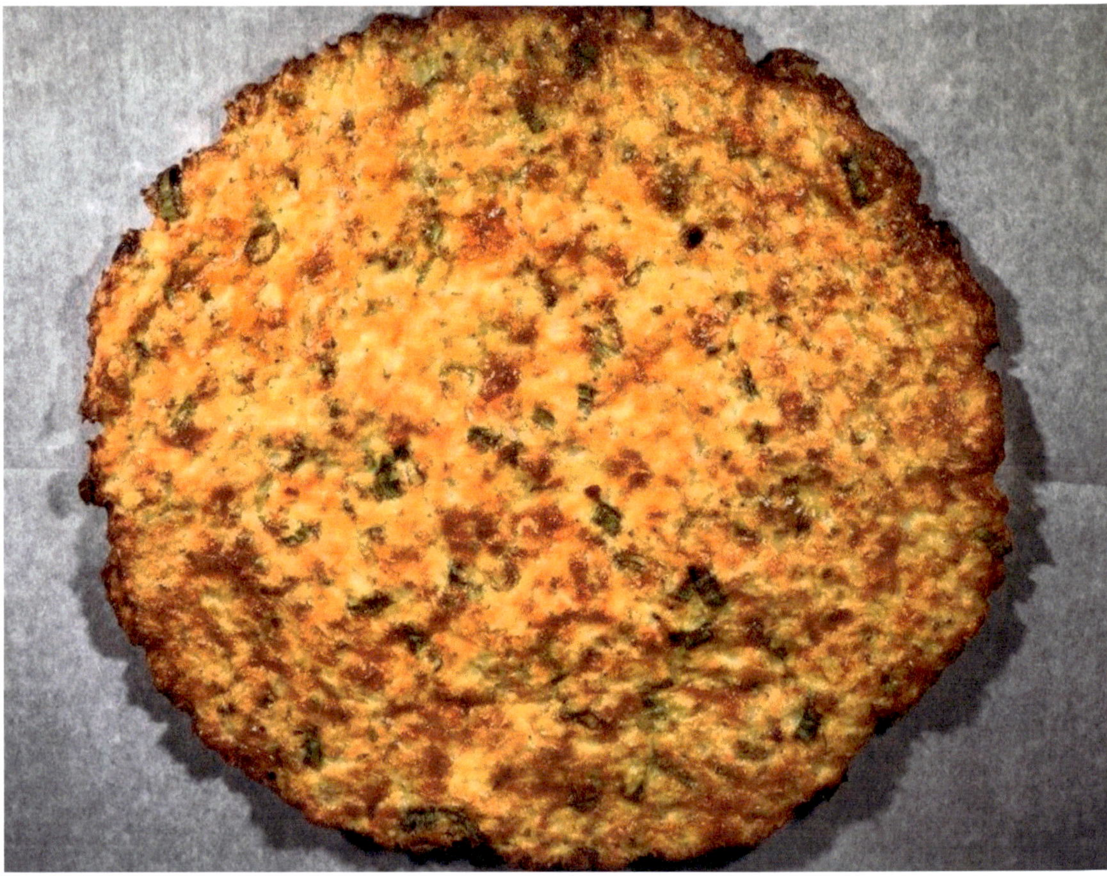

Once your crust has baked until golden brown, remove from the oven and add your desired toppings. Place back into the oven until your cheese has melted.

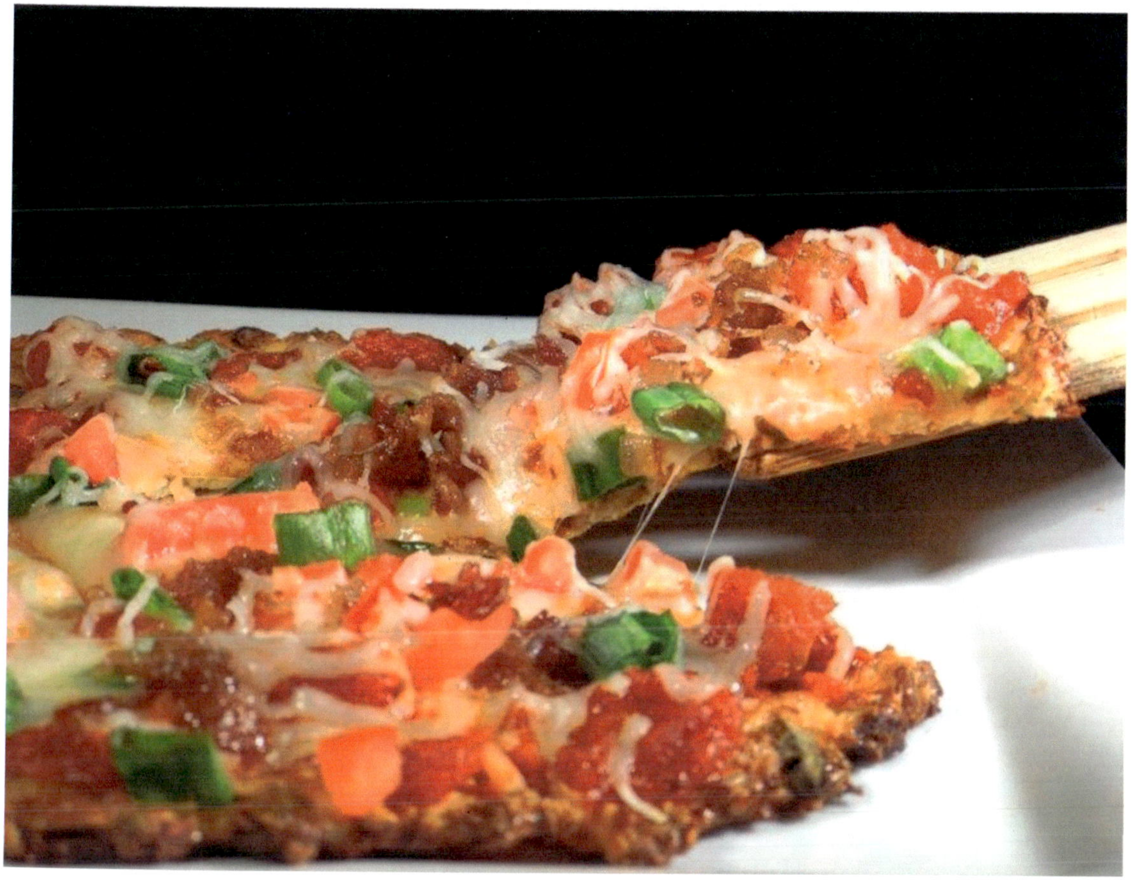

During this demo, I sliced off one end of my finished crust and set it to the side to make sandwich pieces for my sliders. Yes, this same recipe can be used to bake sandwich pieces! Sometimes using lettuce wraps just does not do the trick. Since I do not eat bread, this is a creative way to enjoy a sandwich or a hamburger and still have a similar experience.

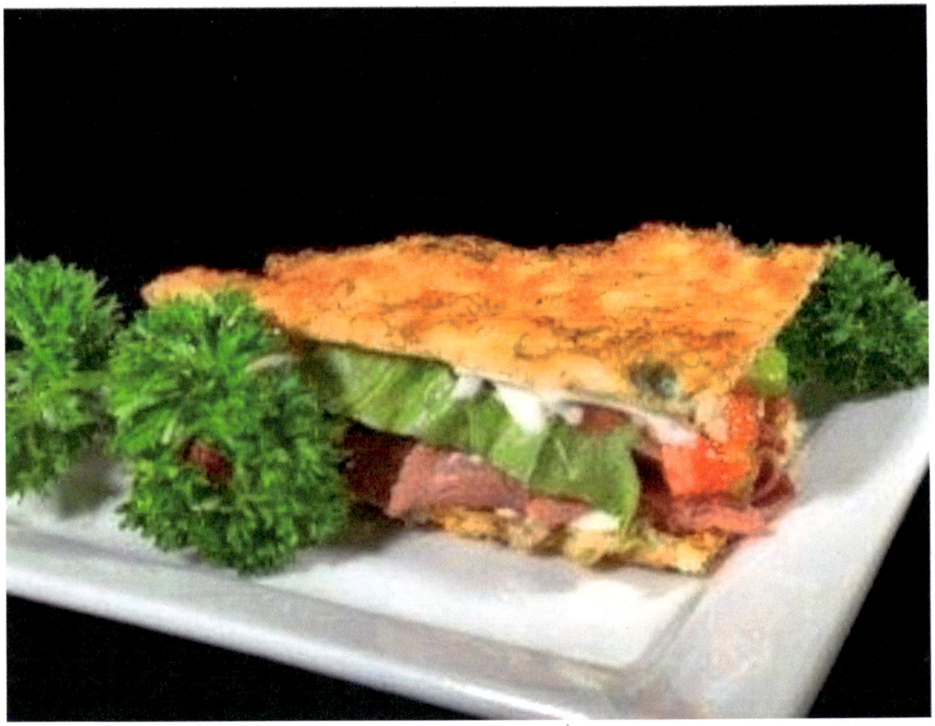

Spaghetti with Spaghetti Squash

There are several substitutions for pasta noodles. Spaghetti squash is one of my favorites. It looks just like pasta! I knew nothing about this little vegetable until a colleague showed me a recipe. Spaghetti squash contains fiber, minerals, and a wide range of vitamins.

The following ingredients were used to complete this recipe:

- 1 pound of ground chicken
- 1 medium sized spaghetti squash
- 2 cups of baby bella mushrooms
- ½ medium sized Vidalia onion (chopped)
- ½ green bell pepper (chopped)
- 1 can of tomato sauce
- 1½ packages of spaghetti seasoning
- white salt (season to taste)
- black pepper (season to taste)
- 2 tablespoons of brown sugar (optional – tones down the tomato)

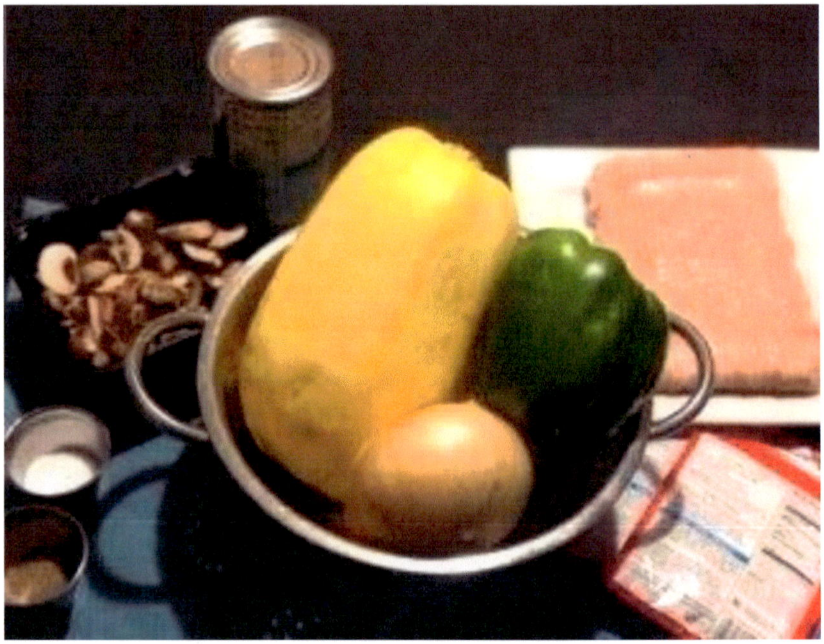

First, you will need to prepare your spaghetti squash since it will take the longest to cook. Preheat oven to 400 degrees. Slice your spaghetti squash in half and remove the seeds. Fill a baking pan with ½ to an inch of water. You can add a little salt to the water if you want or use vegetable broth instead of water. Place the halves with the meat side down in the baking pan. Bake 30-40 minutes.

To prepare your meat sauce, brown your meat of choice with chopped onions, bell peppers, white salt, and black pepper. Add mushrooms to the meat almost when the meat is completed browning. Add the tomato sauce, the pack of spaghetti seasoning and add about 1½ cups of water. As an option, add brown sugar to this sauce. Mix well and let it come to a boil, then simmer for about 15-20 minutes.

Once the spaghetti squash is done, remove from the pan and let it cool for at least 10 minutes. Once it has cooled enough to handle, use a fork to comb the meat out. It will look just like pasta!

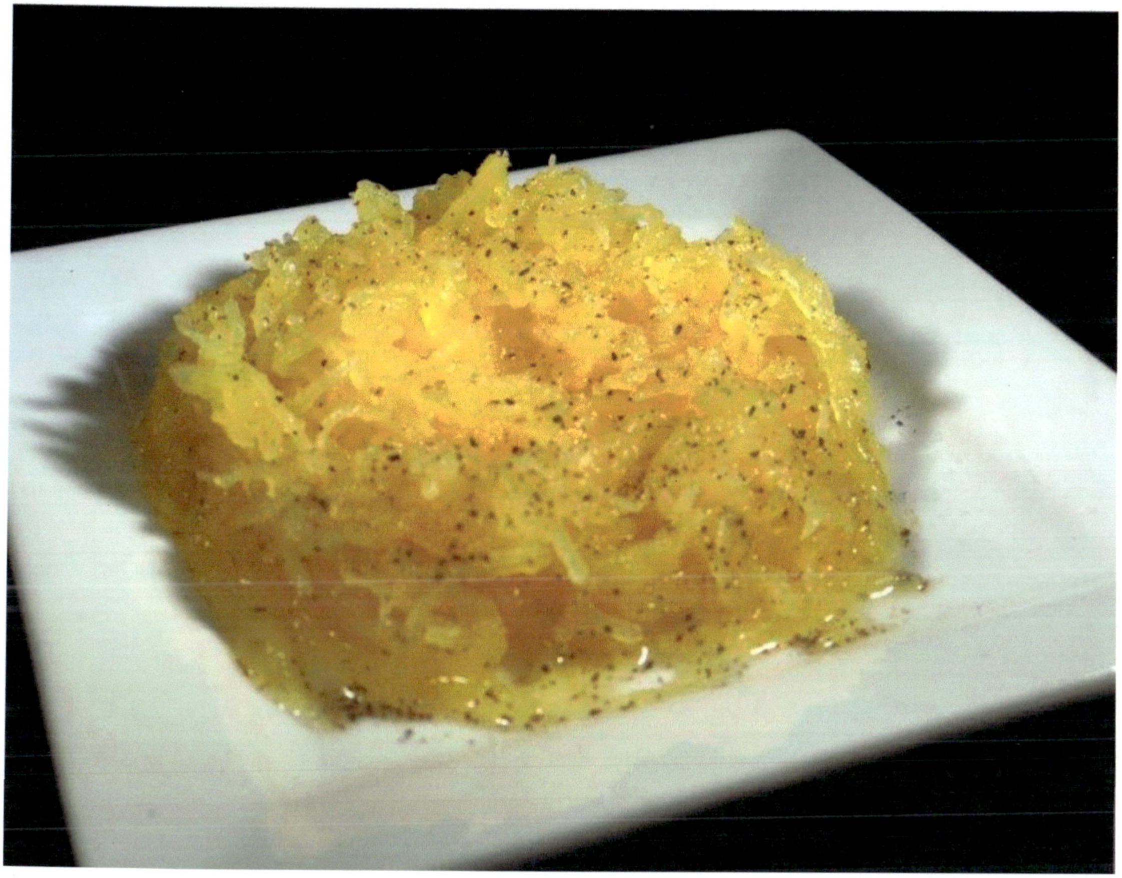

You can either add the squash to the meat sauce or leave separate and add the meat sauce to your plated portion of spaghetti squash. I added a little grated parmesan cheese on the top of my finished dish.

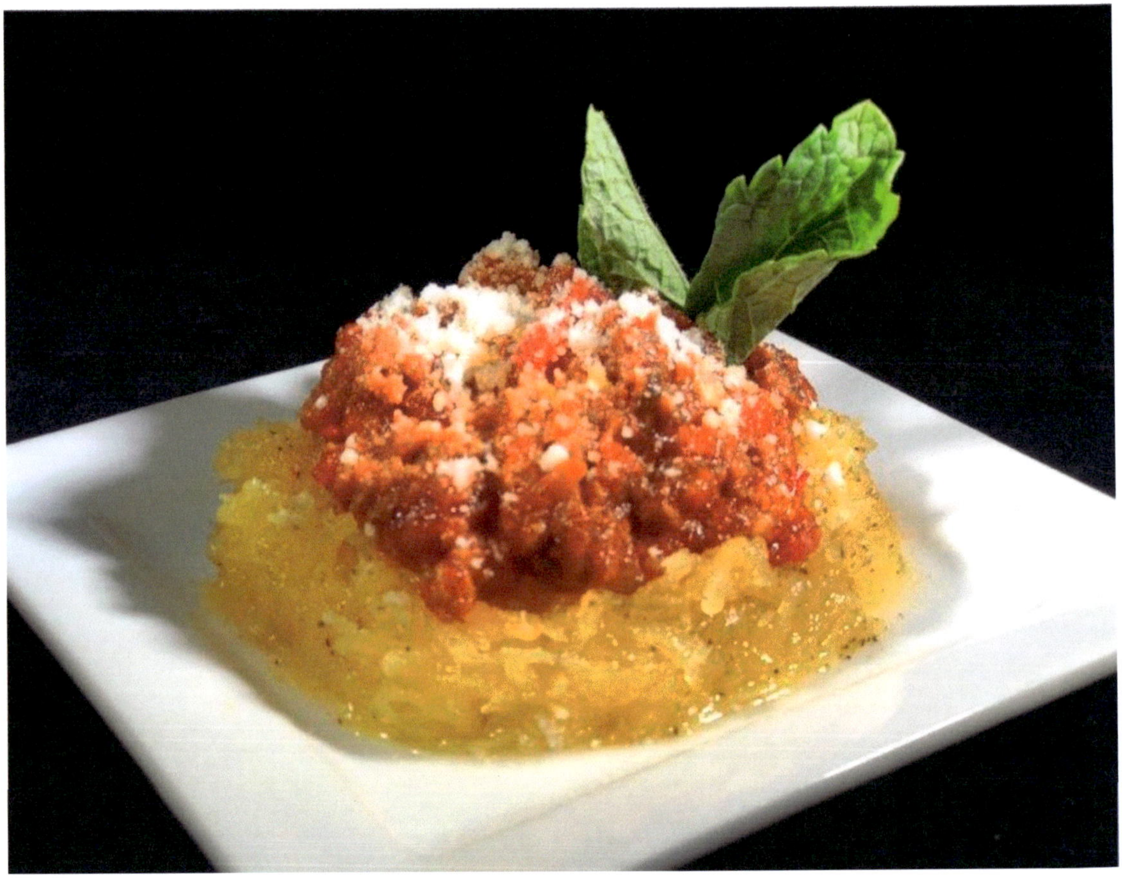

Chicken Salad

I love chicken salad. However, usually I would eat chicken salad with crackers. I learned how to make my own version of this salad with a flavorful combination of ingredients. To substitute the crackers, I eat this salad with black bean chips or I make a cauliflower pizza crust and cut it up to make sandwich pieces.

Make note of the following ingredients:

- 2 cups skinless chicken (skinless chicken legs were used)
- ½ cup of chopped Vidalia onion
- ½ cup of chopped green onion
- ¼ cup turkey bacon bits
- ½ cup of sundried tomatoes
- 1 cup of mayonnaise
- ¼ teaspoon white salt
- ¼ teaspoon black pepper
- zesty herb seasoning

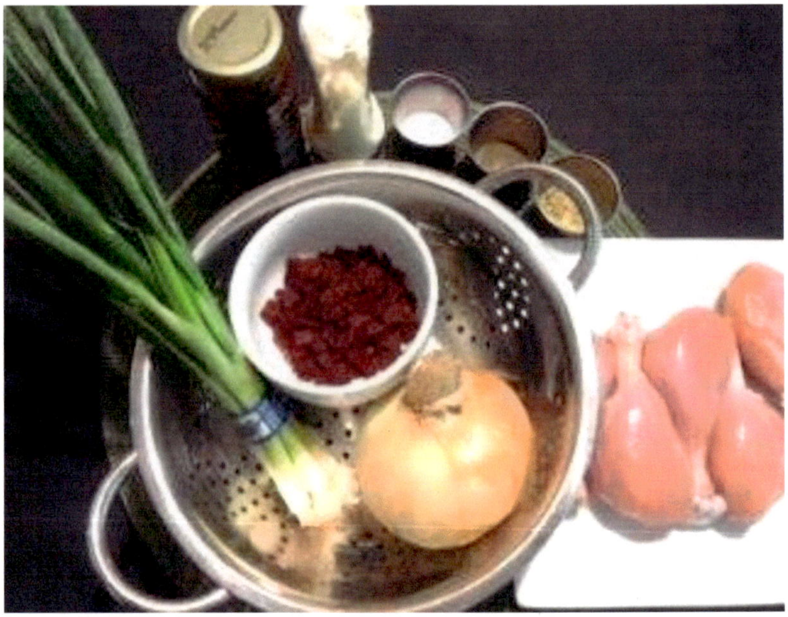

Preheat oven to 350 degrees.

Wash your chicken and place in baking dish. Season chicken with a little white salt, black pepper, and zesty herb seasoning. Add a little extra virgin olive oil and onions across the top of the chicken.

Bake the chicken. Baking time varies. I bake mine for about an hour.

Once the chicken is done, let it cool for at least 15 minutes. After it has cooled enough to handle, chop into pieces or shred using fork and add to bowl.

Mix the chopped/shredded chicken with the turkey bacon bits, chopped sundried tomatoes, chopped green onions, and mayonnaise. You may want to add a pinch of white salt and black pepper. You can use a healthier version of mayonnaise though it is a little more expensive.

With black bean chips:

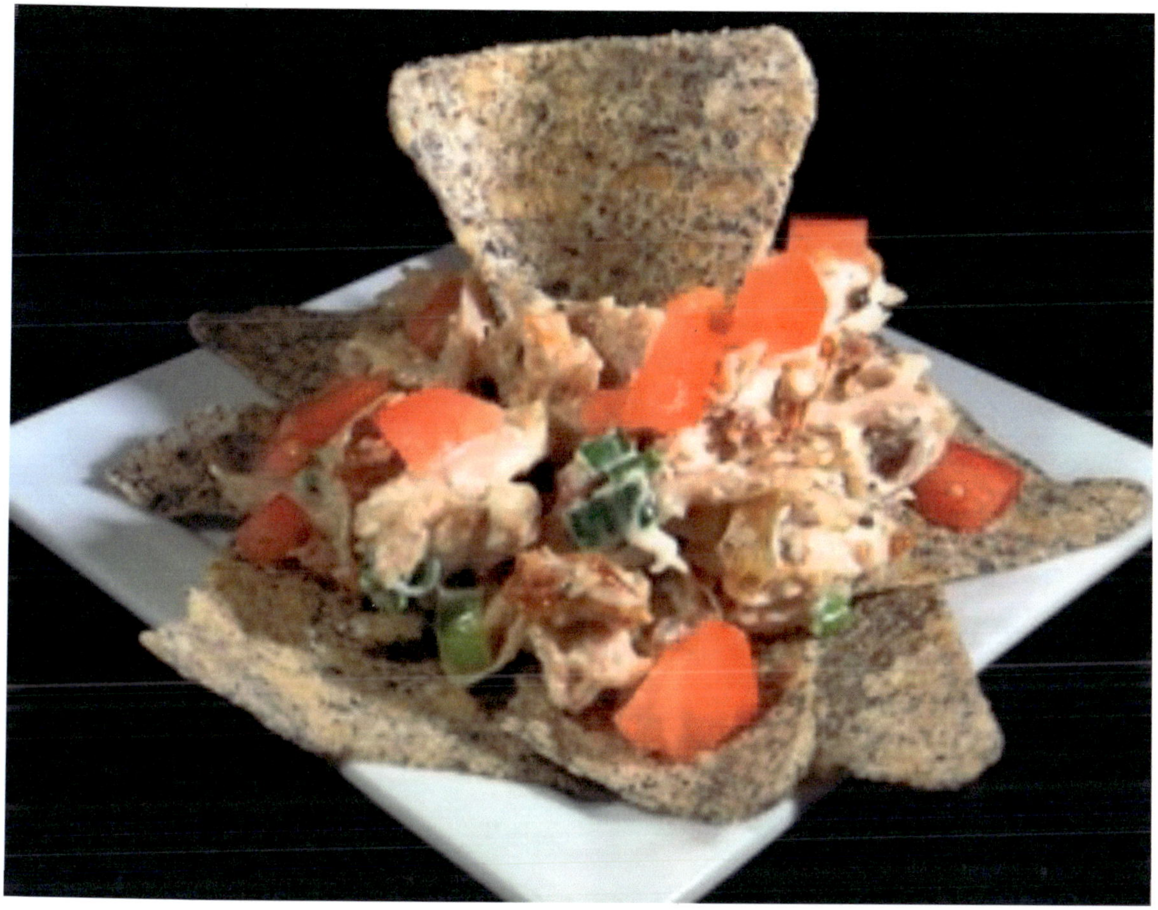

With cauliflower pizza crust sandwich pieces:

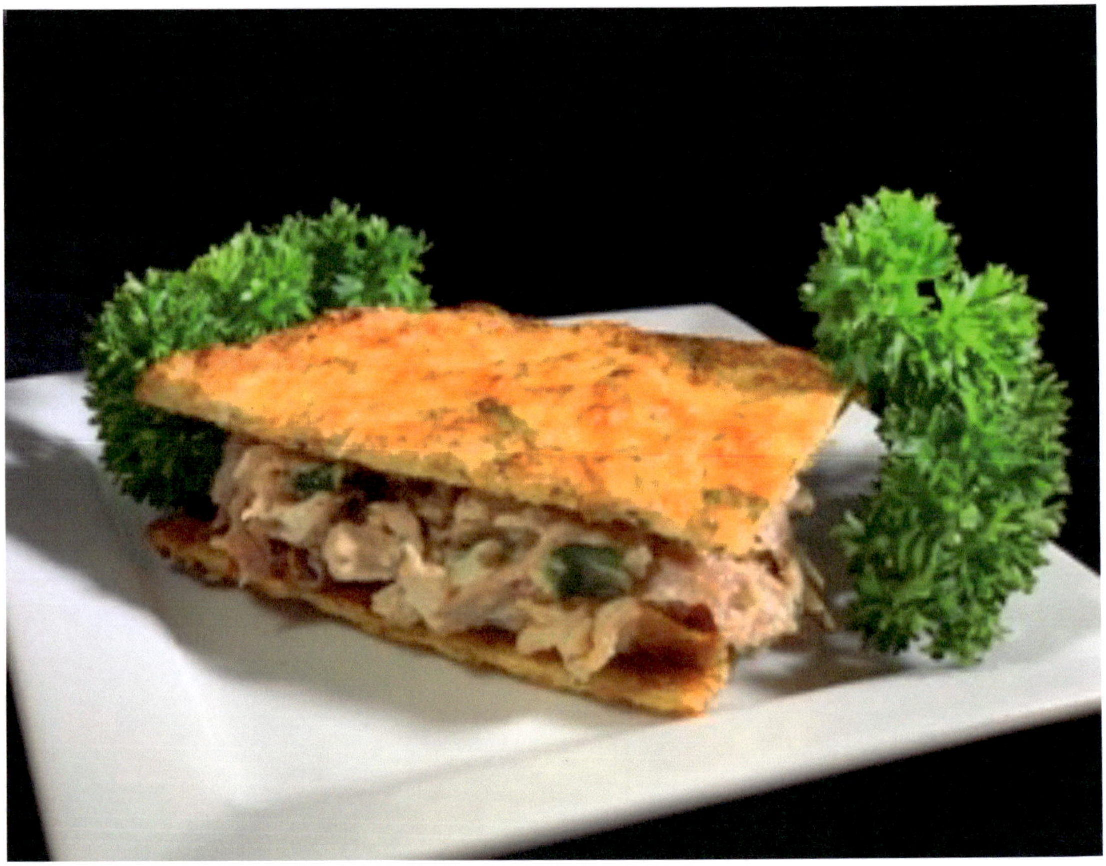

Food For Thought NUMBer 3...

My mother has been a diabetic for at least 15 years. About 4 years ago, she was placed on insulin along with taking the Metformin pills. She has taken on some of my recent eating habits such as cutting down on eating starches. It has been a long while since I've seen her eat white potatoes and she can cook a mean dish of home fried potatoes! I am pleased to report as of July 2018, her doctor has taken her off insulin.

Last Mother's Day, the following was inscribed inside the card: Daughter, you amaze me. You inspire me. And you make me incredibly proud. I am truly humbled to be an inspiration to my mother. Through God, I can do all things and be amazing.

Berries – The Health Benefits

Fruit is not a diabetic's friend. They contain sugars. The over consumption of carbohydrates and sugars is what negatively affects the function of your pancreas. Over time, the pancreas will stop functioning normally and naturally producing the insulin our bodies need. Some groups of fruit contain more sugar than others. Berries are known as a "superfood" for diabetics. Berries are packed with vitamins, antioxidants, and fiber. As a bonus, they are low in the glycemic index (how slow or quickly they increase blood glucose levels). There are recommended portions to consider. The recommended portions for blackberries, blueberries, and raspberries are ¾ cup and strawberries, 1½ cup.

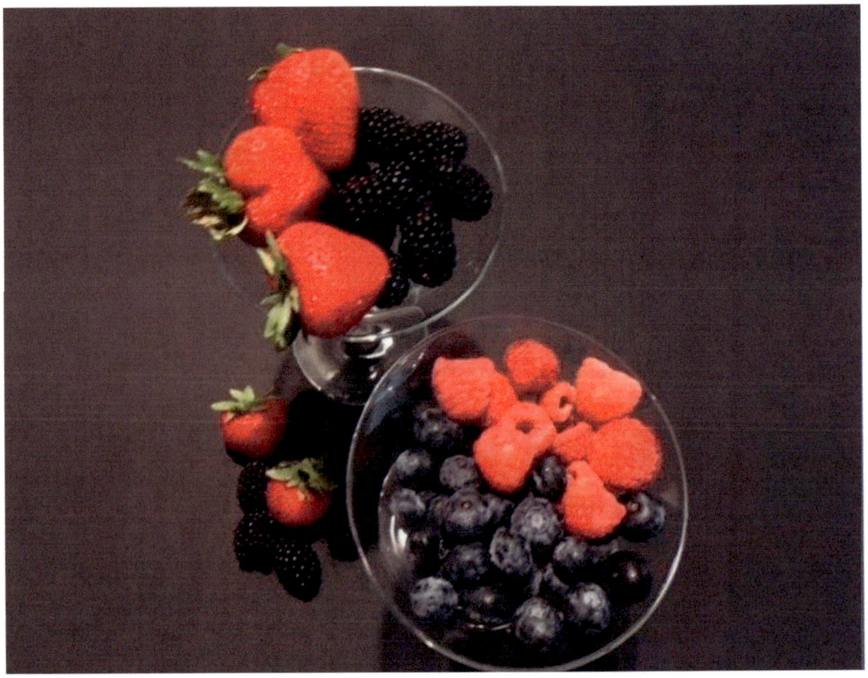

Zucchini, Vidalia Onion, and Bell Pepper Stir Fry

I love this combination of vegetables; they complement each other with both presenta-tion and flavor. You can stir fry on the stove or grill.

You will need the following:

- 3 – 4 nice sized zucchini
- ½ Vidalia onion sliced
- ½ bell pepper (Red was used. You also use a combination of the yellow, red, and orange.)
- white salt
- black pepper
- zesty herb seasoning
- butter

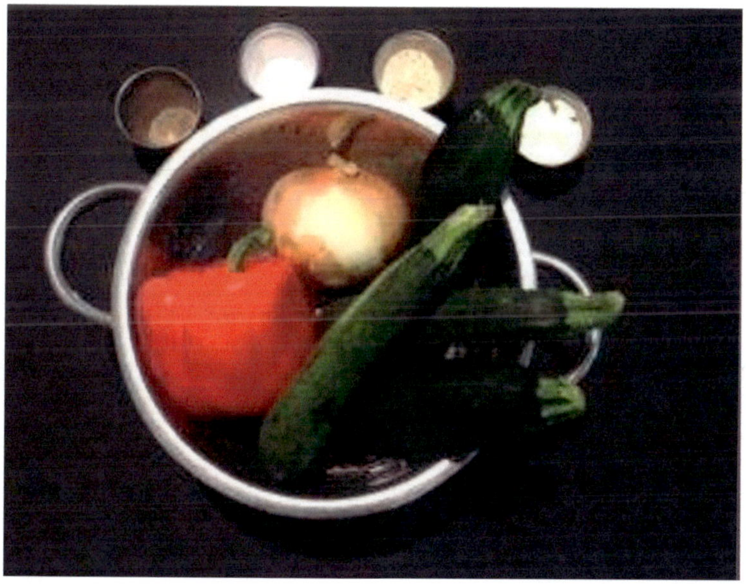

Slice all of your vegetables and place in a bowl. Add at least 2 tablespoons of butter. Season with white salt, black pepper, and zesty herb. Season to taste.

Mix by hand or spoon until the combination of vegetables, seasoning, and butter are well blended.

If you are grilling, try not to cook directly over the coals. Grill until the onions are slightly caramelized. If using a pan to stir fry, stir-fry until onions are slightly caramelized. That is it!

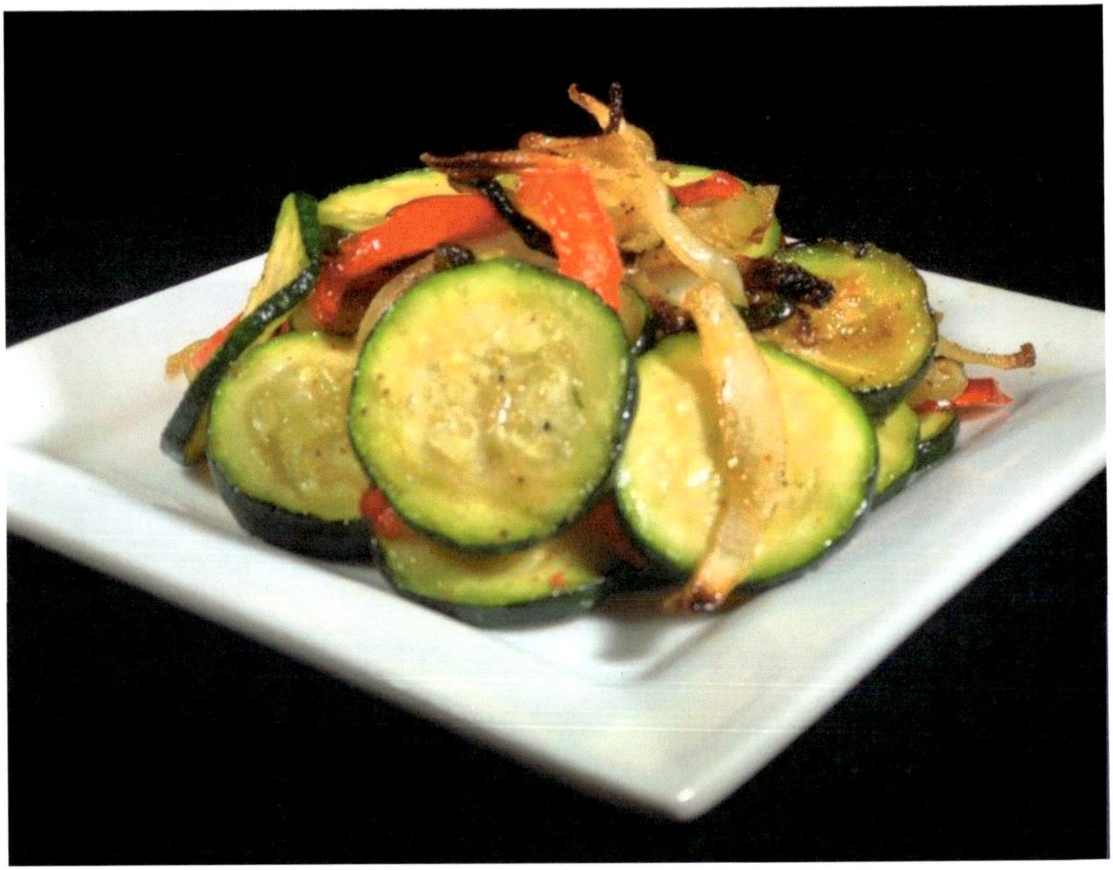

Mashed Sweet Potatoes

I have a confession. I am not a fan of sweet potatoes. I love sweet potato pie. I know. You are wondering, *'How can this be?'* Well, it is a fact. I have had to adapt to eating sweet potato fries when I get that craving for french fries dipped in tartar sauce. Only those from Seattle, Washington will understand that combination. I have found a compromise for sweet potato pie. My mashed sweet potatoes are sweetened with brown sugar Splenda.

The following items are needed for this dish:

- 1 medium sized sweet potato
- 2 tablespoons of butter (unsalted)
- 1 teaspoon of cinnamon
- 1 teaspoon of nutmeg
- ¼ teaspoon of white salt
- ½ teaspoon Vanilla Extract
- 1 tablespoon of brown sugar Splenda
- ¼ cup of 2% milk

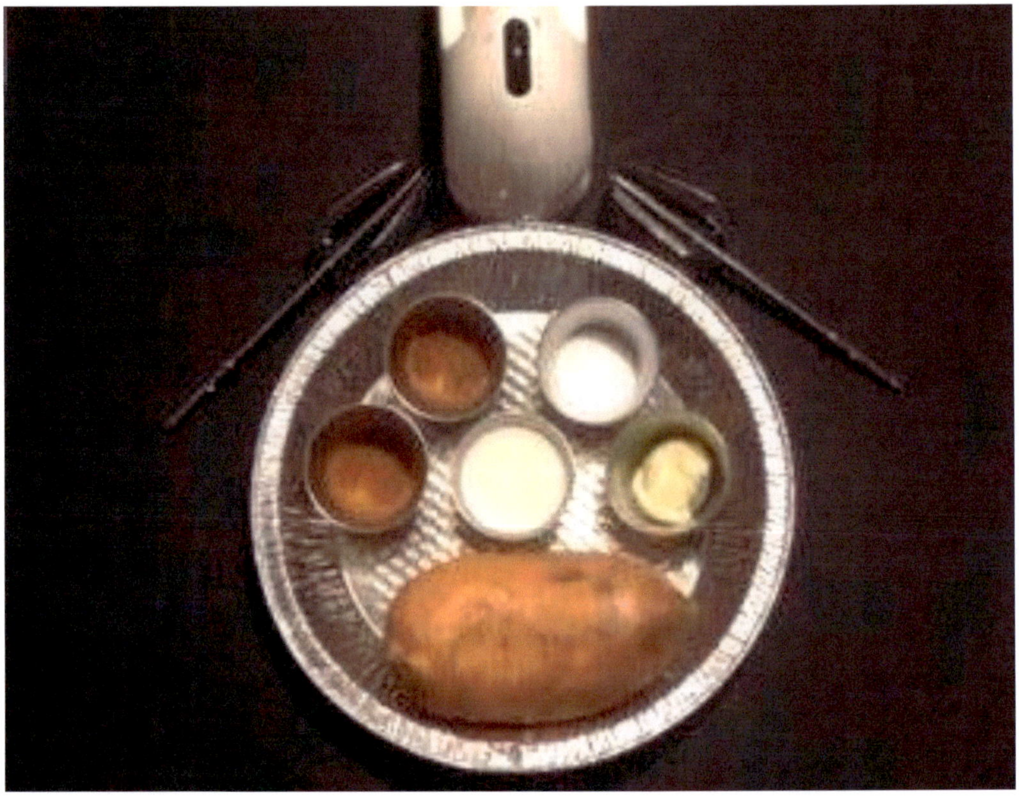

Preheat oven to 350 degrees.

Place sweet potato in a baking dish and bake for approximately 45 minutes. Once potato is done, take out of the oven and let cool. It needs to be cooled enough to allow the skin to be peeled. Place peeled sweet potato in a bowl. Add butter, cinnamon, nutmeg, salt, brown sugar Splenda, and milk. Use a mixing spoon to evenly combine. Use hand mixer to blend the ingredients. I prefer mine chilled.

The completed dish is a delicious compromise to the sinful sweet potato pie.

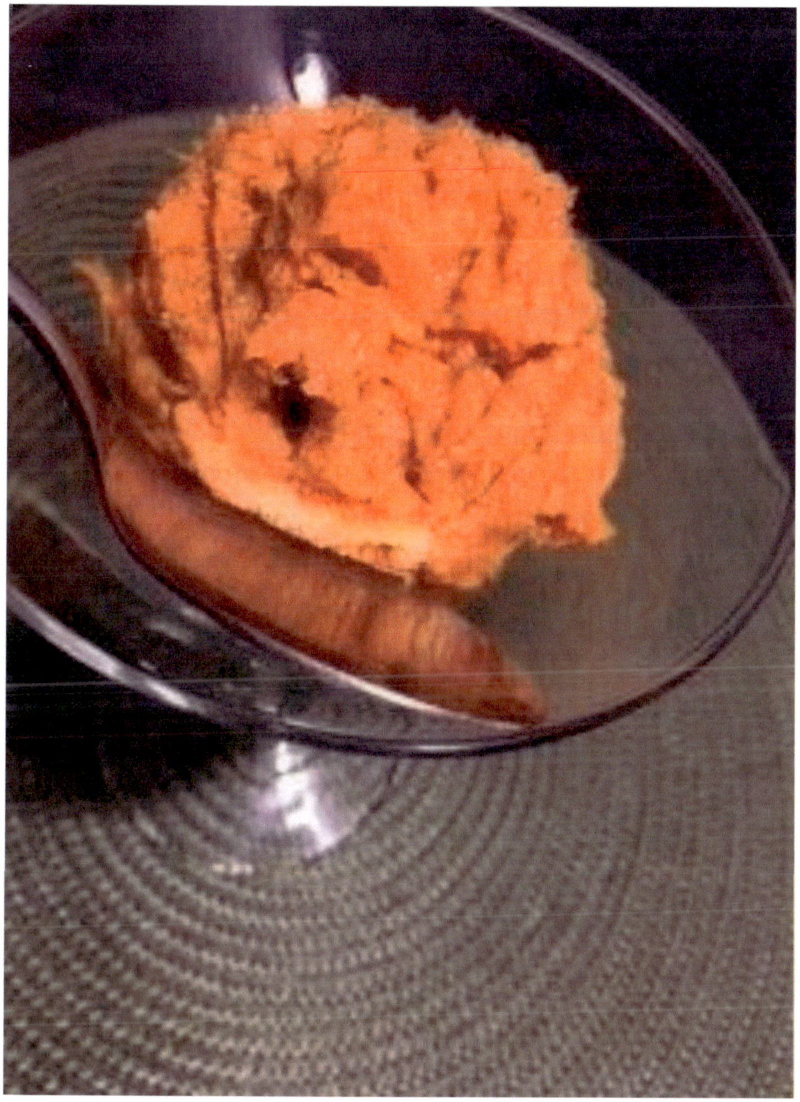

Chicken Fajita Cobb Salad

A salad can be an entire meal in a bowl. There are so many creative combinations of vegetables, fruit, and meat to make this lettuce based meal a healthy and satisfying lunch and/or dinner dish. I have fallen in food lust with one combination!

My best friend took me to a Mexican restaurant for my birthday. Since my diet is limited, I chose to order one of their salads. It was a Chicken Fajita Cobb Salad. The ingredients included mixed salad greens (not iceberg lettuce), grilled chicken, black beans, sliced avocado, queso fresco cheese, bacon bits, diced tomato, roasted corn, and tortilla strips. I asked them to hold the corn and the tortilla strips. For the dressing, I chose the Chipotle Ranch, which is freshly made at the restaurant. All I can say is, "Freaking amazing!"

I had to include this wonderful masterpiece in my recipe suggestions. Usually at restaurants, they give you all of this lettuce and fudge on the other ingredients. But this salad had a taste of everything in each bite!

You will need the following:

- lettuce greens (pictured is red leaf lettuce)
- tomatoes
- avocado
- lime juice (add to avocado slices to keep them from browning)
- bacon bits
- black beans
- queso fresco cheese
- grilled chicken
- dressing of your choice

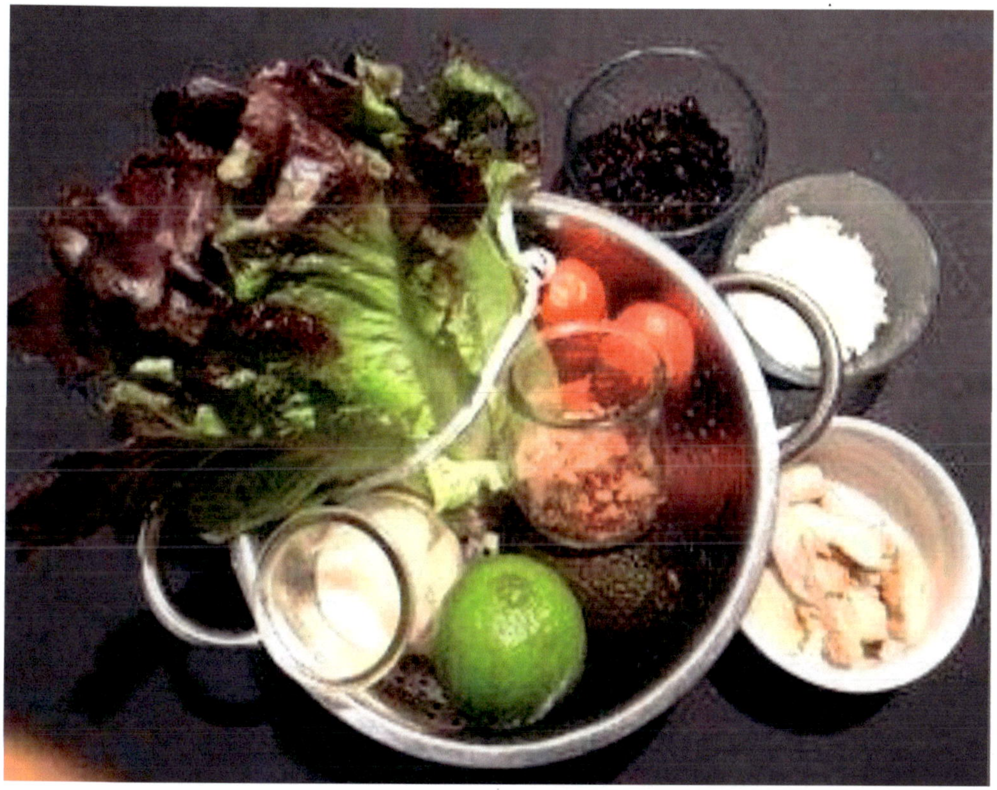

I did not provide measurements for this salad on purpose. There is no mixing or seasoning to do, just slicing and chopping. I made this dish diabetic-friendly by leaving off the corn and the tortilla strips. You can add crispy onions or some black bean chips if you want that crunch. Below, I have mimicked the presentation of the salad served.

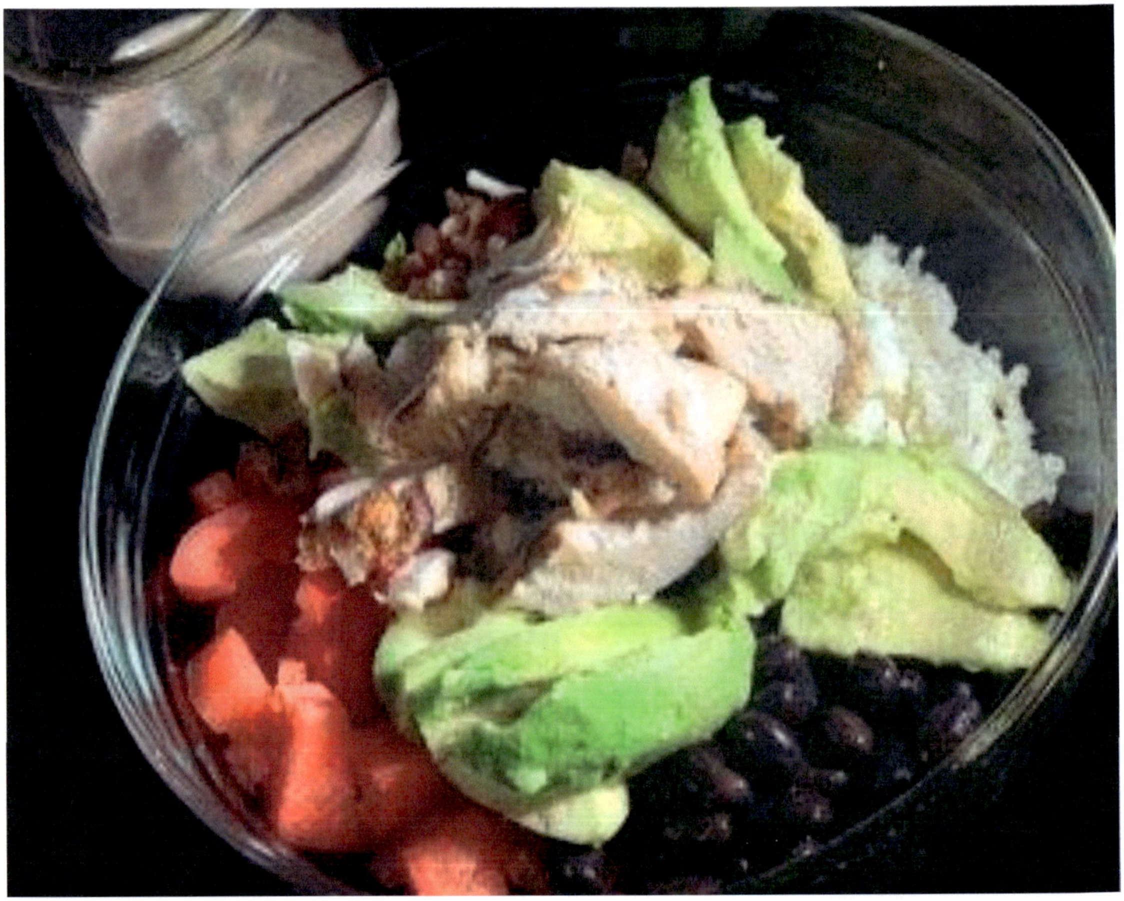

FEATURED

Brownies Made with Avocados

Can we talk about this one? You have no idea how much pull back I received in the beginning when I spoke about these wonderful chocolate delights. Avocados... chocolate... brownies...WHAT!?! That doesn't even sound right. However, when I cooked a batch and allowed everyone to sample them, I received so many requests for the recipe it had to be the featured recipe of this book. No flour. Period. They bake and taste like brownies made the traditional way.

You will need the following items:

- ¾ cup of ripe avocados
- ¼ lime (I do not want my avocados to brown)
- 2 large eggs
- 1 full stick of melted butter (unsalted)
- 3-4 tablespoons of Nut butter (I used sunflower butter)
- ½ teaspoon baking soda
- ¼ teaspoon white salt
- ⅓ cup of brown sugar Splenda + 1 tablespoon of regular Splenda
- ⅓ cup cocoa powder (unsweetened)
- ¼ ounce of unsweetened Baker's Chocolate bar melted
- ⅓ cup dark chocolate chips (semi-sweet to top your brownies)
- parchment paper

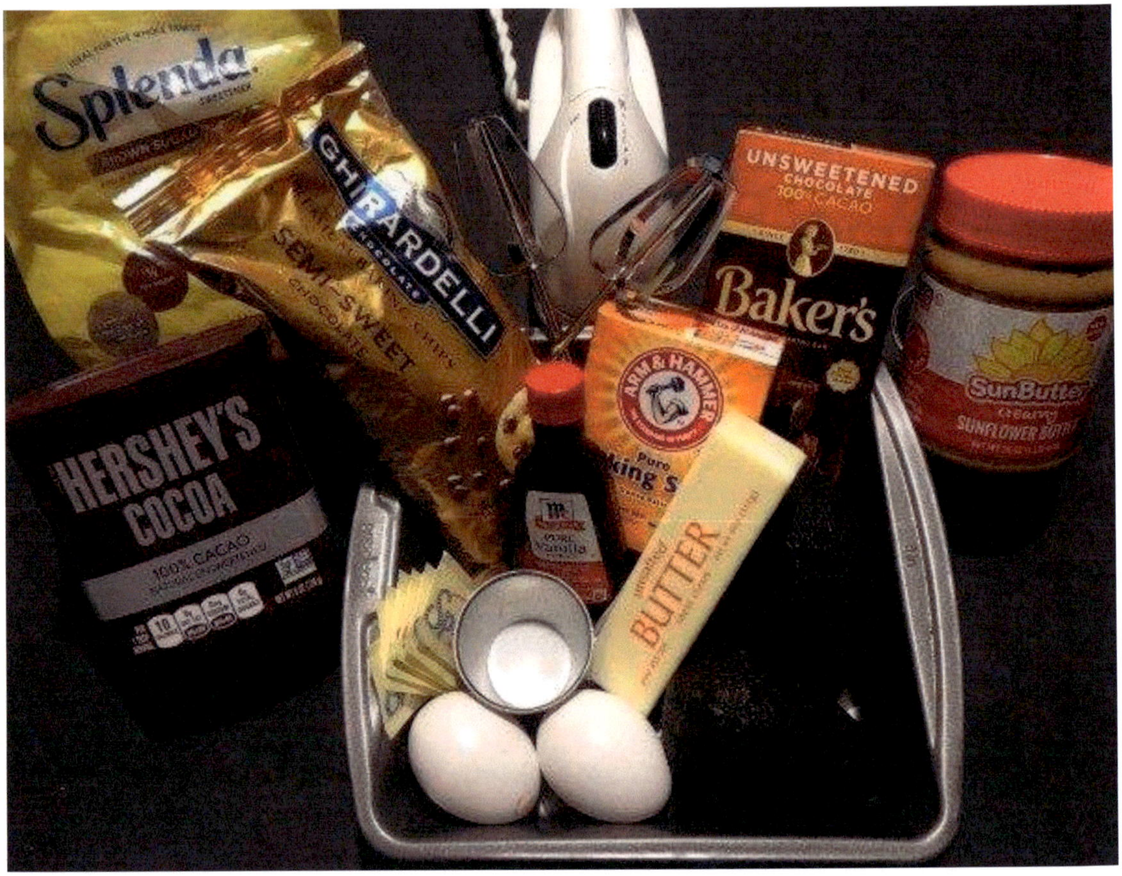

Preheat oven to 350 degrees.

Let's start with melting your ¼ ounce of Baker's Chocolate bar.

Fill a small pot with about 2 cups of water. Place the piece of chocolate bar in a dish that can fit over the pan (I used a pie pan). Boil the water on medium. Remove from heat once melted.

Melt butter in a microwave safe dish for less than 30 seconds.

Half your avocados, take the seed out, and scoop the meat out with a spoon. Take half of the lime and squeeze the juice over the avocados (you only need about a tablespoon of the juice).

Mash the avocado with a spoon and try to get it a smooth as you can. You can use a food processor; however, you will not need it for more than 30 seconds.

After you have smoothed the avocado, add all of the other ingredients except for the semi-sweet chocolate chips.

I used a hand mixer on the speed of 2. Mix initially for about 10 seconds. Stir your mixture and mix again for about 15 seconds. Do not over mix. Less than 30 seconds is perfect.

Line a small baking pan with parchment paper and spoon brownie mix into the pan. Sprinkle your semi-sweet chocolate chips over the top.

Bake for approximately 25 minutes.

Allow to cool for at least an hour. When you take them out, they will be a little spongy. Once they cool and settle, they will have the right texture.

I guarantee these will blow you away. I am not a chocolate lover. I sampled a few pieces when they were done and kept testing to make sure my mouth wasn't playing tricks on me.

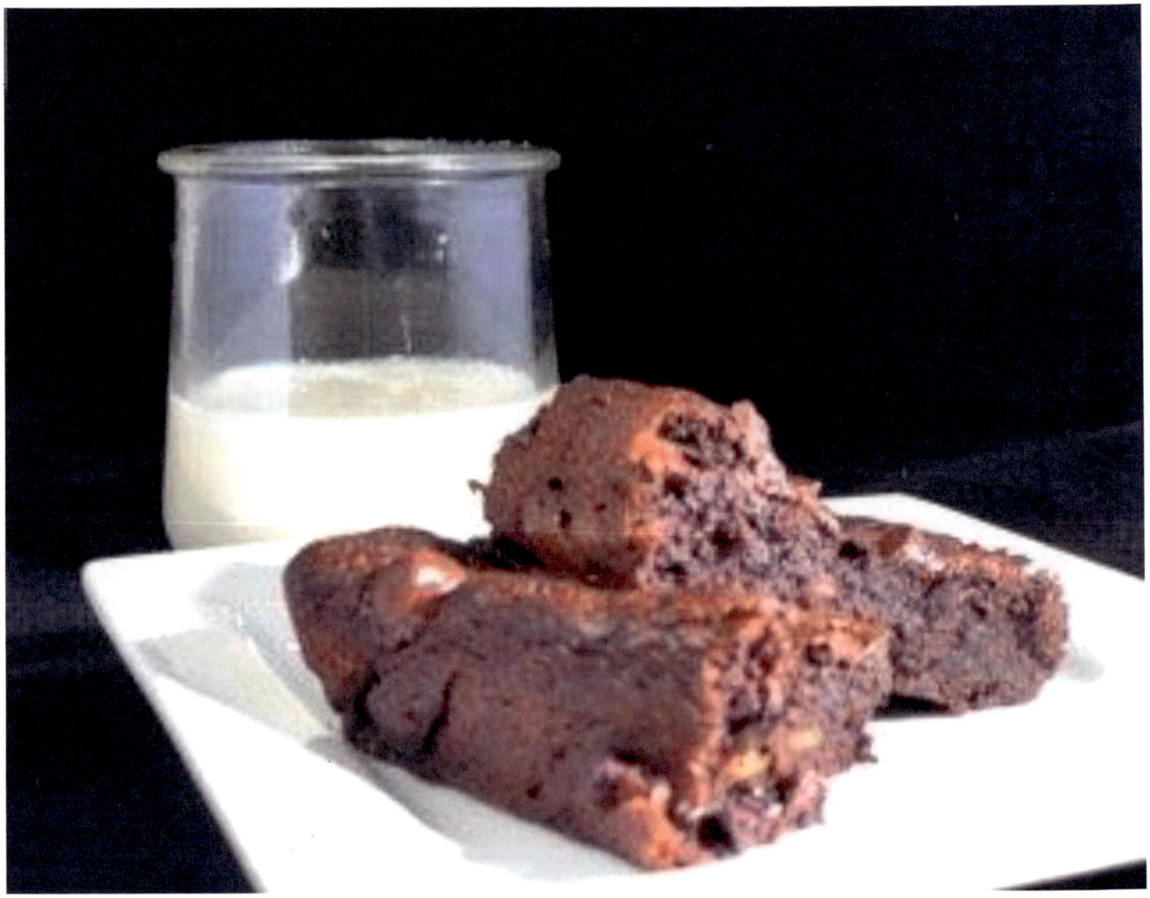

Zucchini Lasagna

Don't judge me...I never know how to cook lasagna until experimenting with recipes for this book. All of these years, I did not realize what I was missing out on. I came about this recipe after going on a cruise for the Christmas holiday in 2017. They served this lasagna made with zucchini and eggplant instead of noodles one night at dinner and it was amazing. They only served it one night and I was so disappointed. The recipe that follows is just with the zucchini, not the eggplant. You can also use cabbage or spinach leaves as a substitute. If using cabbage, make sure you use leaves from the second or third layer that are a little more tender and boil them first. Cabbage can be a tough layer separator.

You will need the following:

- 1 pound of ground meat of choice (pictured is ground beef)
- 2 medium cloves of garlic
- ¼ cup of chopped Vidalia onions
- 1 teaspoon of white salt
- 1 teaspoon of black pepper
- 1 teaspoon dried oregano
- ¼ cup of chopped green onions
- ½ cup grated parmesan
- 1 (16 ounce) package of cottage cheese
- 1-2 medium to large zucchinis
- 1 jar of marinara sauce (Bertolli brand marinara with burgundy wine sauce pictured)
- 2 cups grated mozzarella cheese

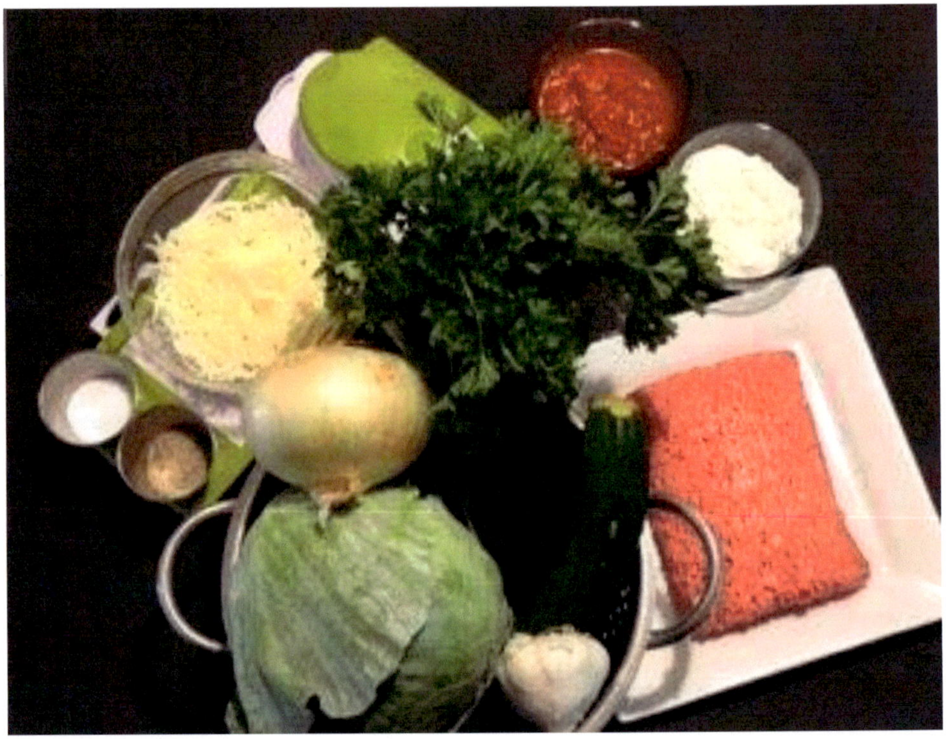

Using a slicer, slice zucchini into around 16 semi thin pieces. Line a cookie sheet or flat dish with paper towels. Place zucchini slices on the paper towel. Salt each side and let stand for 15-20 minutes. This step is very important. Zucchini contains water. This process will help extract the water out of the vegetable. You can also use a tabletop grill in place of this method. The object is to extract the water so your lasagna will not be watery.

Preheat your oven to 350 degrees.

In a pan, brown your meat adding chopped garlic, chopped Vidalia onion, salt pepper, and oregano.

For the white sauce, I use cottage cheese. In a bowl, mix cottage cheese, green onion, and about ¼ cup of your grated parmesan cheese. Set to the side.

I do not mix the marinara with the meat; but, you can because it is going to mix anyway.

In a medium casserole baking pan, let's start our layers. The first layer is the marinara sauce. Second layer, half of your meat. Third layer, about 8 zucchini slices. Next, scoop half of your cottage cheese mixture then 1 cup of your mozzarella.

Repeat the steps one more time ending with 1 cup of mozzarella. Sprinkle ¼ cup of chopped green onions to the top.

You will have to bake a little longer than traditional lasagna. Bake for about 35-to-45 minutes.

Please allow this dish to cool before slicing. Add the other ¼ of grated parmesan to the top.

This dish is a delicious compromise.

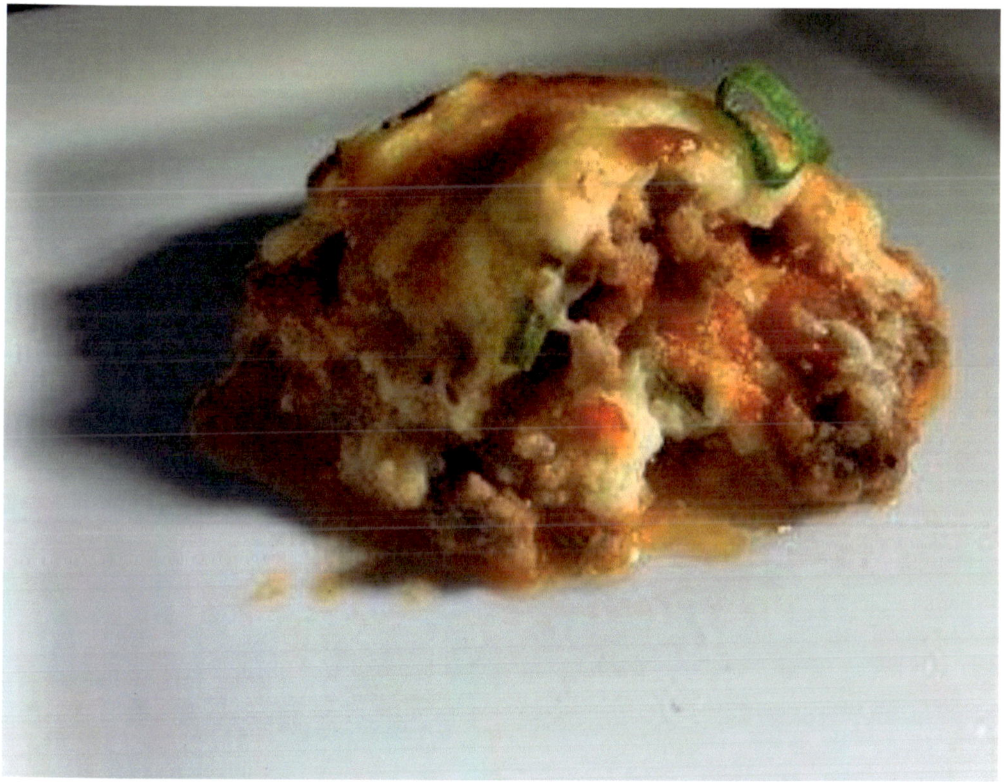

Greek Salad

Once upon a time, I was the secretary of my former subdivision's Home Owners Association (HOA). The president, who was also my neighbor, made a Greek salad for this meeting. I had never heard of a Greek salad. The combination of the vegetables was the bomb.com! I have been hooked on this salad ever since. This salad is light on the ingredients and is a lot leaner than the Fajita Cobb Salad.

You will need the following:

- lettuce (pictured is red leaf)
- sliced tomatoes
- sliced black olives
- sliced red onion
- crumpled feta cheese
- sliced cucumber
- vinaigrette dressing of choice

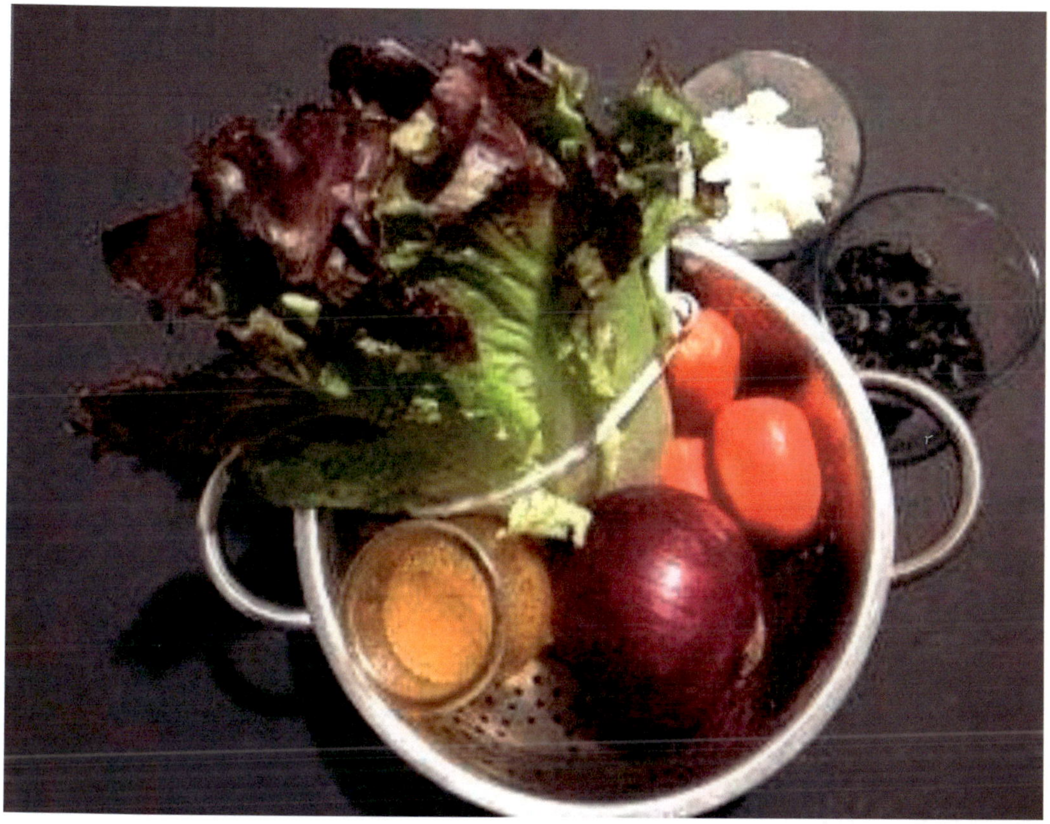

This is another recipe idea that really needs no specific measuring of the ingredients.

Slice your vegetables into your desired portions.

Using lettuce as your base, assemble the other vegetables on the top of the lettuce.

Add salad dressing at the end to prevent the salad from being soggy.

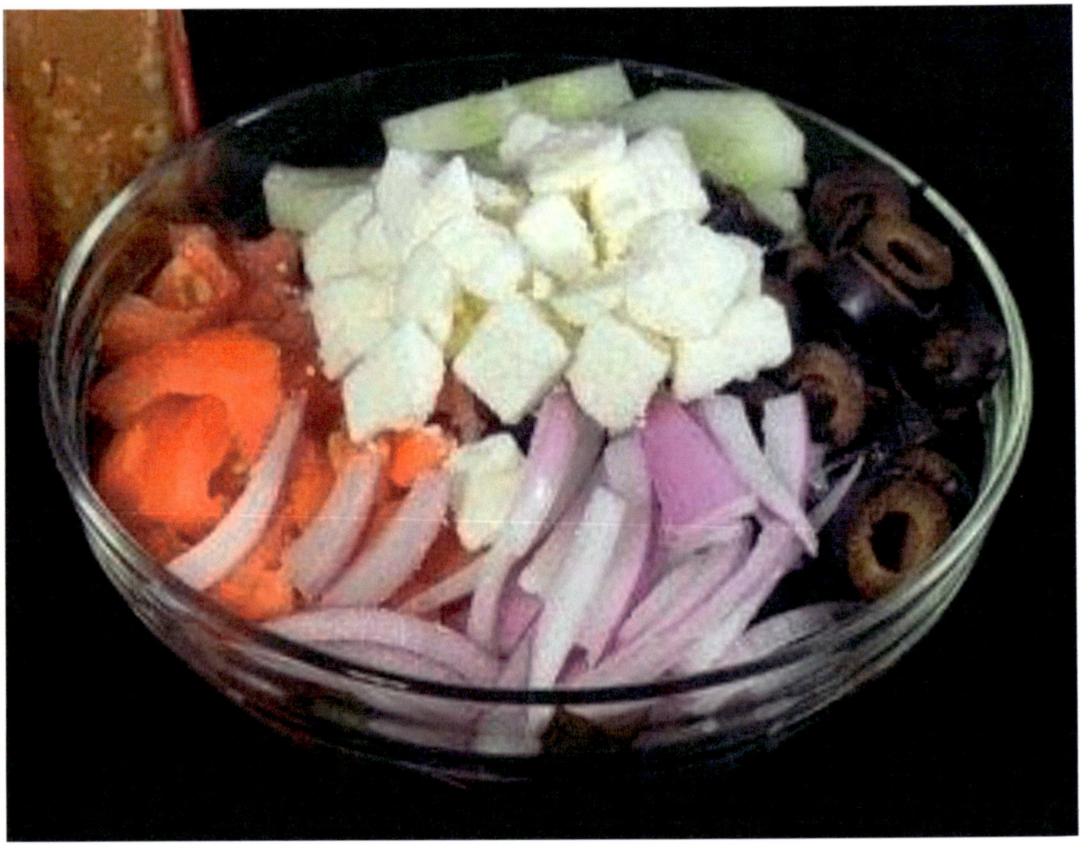

Grilled Chicken, Broccoli, Mushrooms, Onions and Cauliflower Rice in Alfredo Sauce

I was walking down the frozen food aisle in the grocery store and stumbled upon a broccoli and grilled chicken frozen entrée. One of the dishes I do miss is my Chicken Linguine Alfredo. Seeing this entrée gave me the idea of this dish. I cooked it one Sunday and my 16-year-old loved it! This is a delicious compromise.

You will need the following:

- 12 ounces of riced cauliflower (I used a frozen bag found in the frozen food section.)
- 8 ounces of sliced baby bella mushrooms
- 1 (14.5 ounce) jar of Alfredo sauce
- 2 cups of grilled chicken
- ½ cup of sliced Vidalia onions
- 3-4 cups of broccoli
- 1 teaspoon of white salt
- 2-3 tablespoons of extra virgin olive oil
- ½ teaspoon white salt
- ½ teaspoon black pepper
- ½ teaspoon of garlic powder
- cheesecloth or clean dishtowel

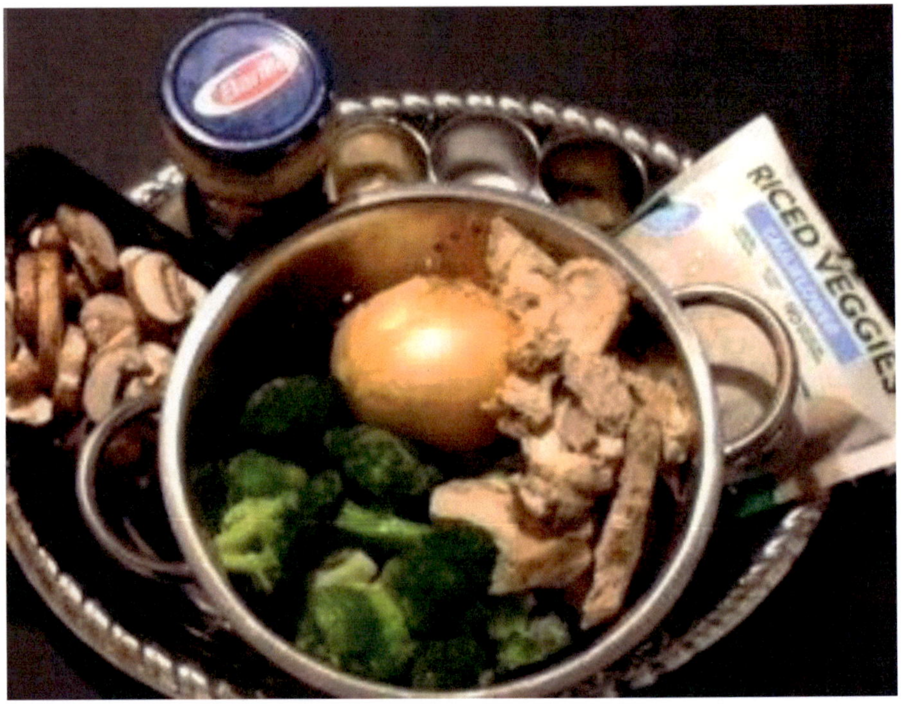

Place the unopened bag of frozen riced cauliflower in the microwave for about 4 minutes to thaw. Open the bag and place the cauliflower in a cheesecloth (or clean dishtowel) and squeeze all of the moisture out. Place to the side.

I also used frozen broccoli and frozen grilled chicken. Of course you can use fresh broccoli and prepare your own grilled or baked chicken. If you are preparing your own chicken, make that item the first task. Place your broccoli and chicken to the side.

In a large skillet, add 2-3 tablespoons of extra virgin olive oil and heat using medium heat. Add the sliced onion and sauté until slightly softened. Add mushrooms and sauté until onions are caramelized and the mushrooms have cooked down. Add the riced cauliflower to the mushrooms and onions and stir fry for about 5 minutes. Add the broccoli and chicken, then the salt, pepper, and garlic powder. Lower the heat and cover. Allow to cook for another 5 minutes.

If you want to leave out the Alfredo sauce, you can. The following picture is without the Alfredo sauce.

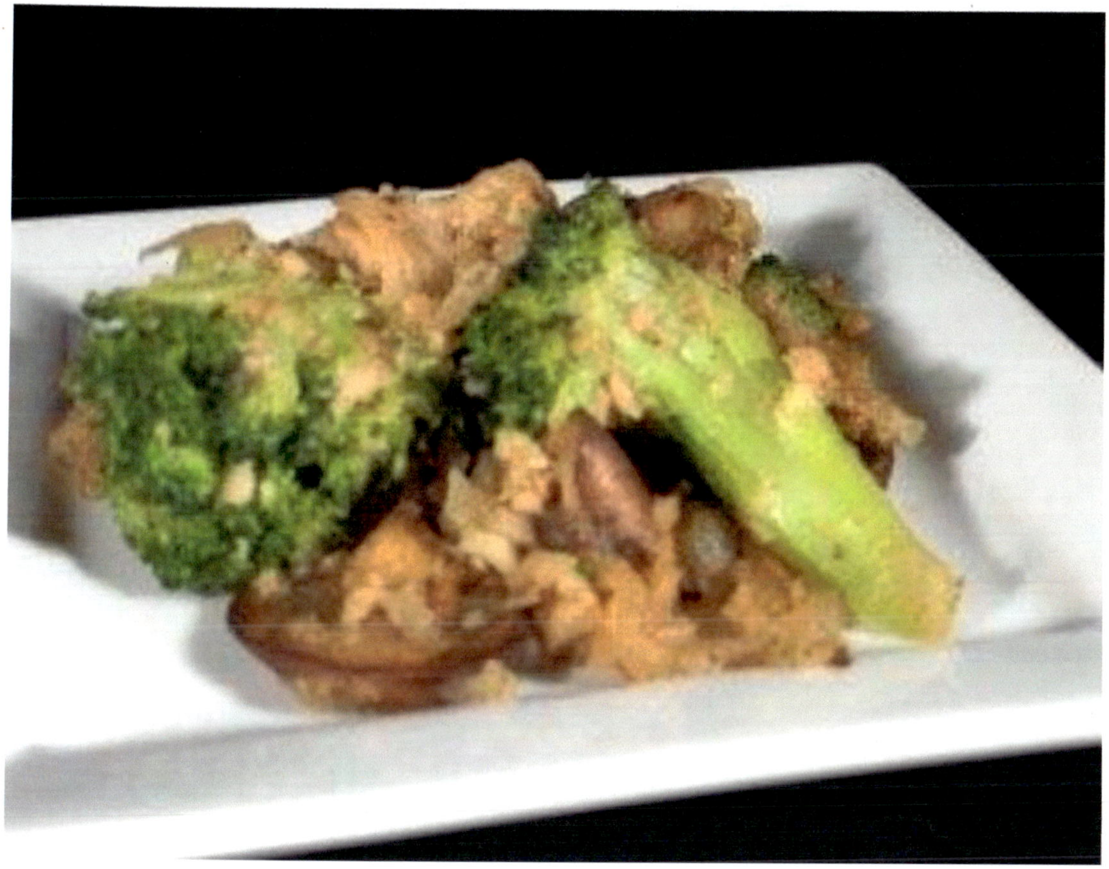

The final step is to add the Alfredo sauce to the dish. Allow to cook another 3-5 minutes covered. My youngest son loves this dish. Pictured is with the Alfredo sauce.

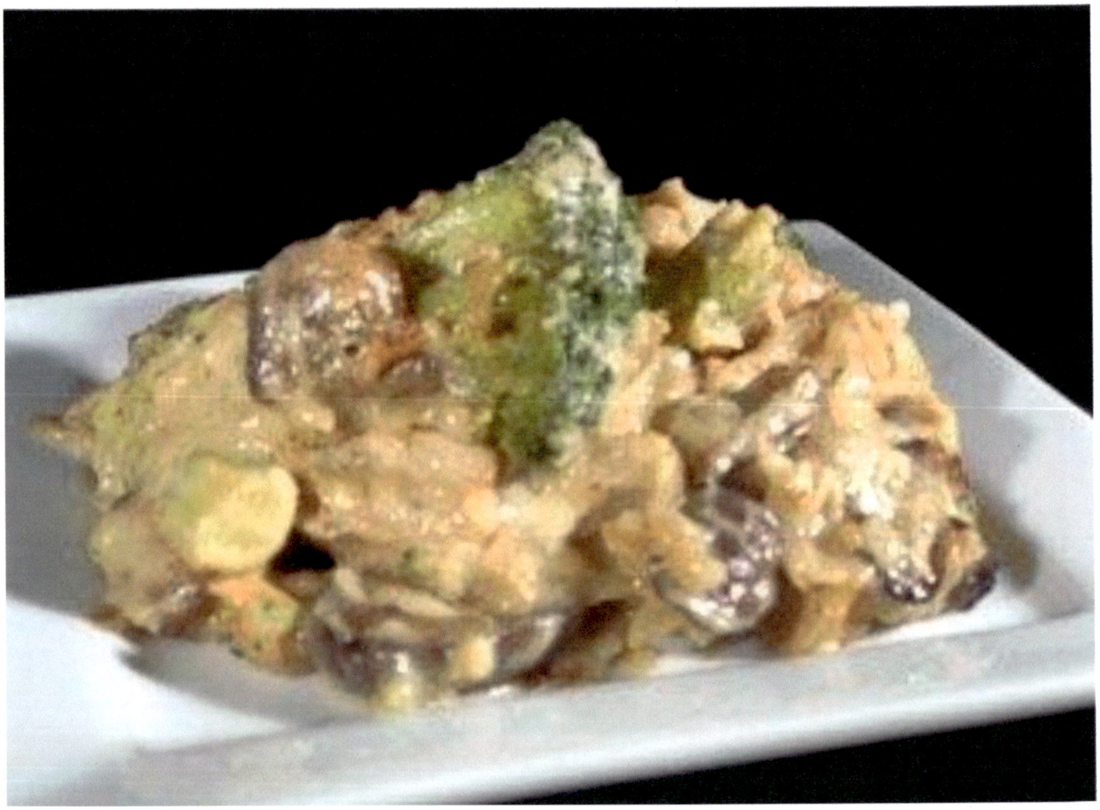

Meatloaf Cake

I know. You are like, *'What?'* Yes. This is a true winner. This is such a creative way to incorporate an entire meal into a unique and fun dish. My version is diabetic-friendly. Instead of mashed potatoes, I used mashed cauliflower. I also used turkey bacon bits instead of pork bacon bits.

The following items are needed:

- 1 pound ground meat (Pictured is ground sirloin)
- 1 large egg
- ½ cup chopped Vidalia onions
- ½ cup chopped green bell pepper
- ½ cup of tomato sauce
- 1 package of McCormick brand meatloaf seasoning (If you do not want to use the seasoning pack, you will need 3 cloves of garlic, ¼ teaspoon of white salt, ¼ teaspoon black pepper, ¼ teaspoon of garlic powder, and ¼ teaspoon of onion powder)
- 1 (8.5 ounce) can of green peas
- 1 (12 ounce) package of frozen mashed cauliflower (Birds Eye brand used – Sour cream and chives)
- 1 cup of bacon bits (pictured is turkey bacon bits)
- 2 cups crispy onions
- ½ Slice of toasted honey wheat bread (crumpled into tiny pieces)
- 2 mini cake pans

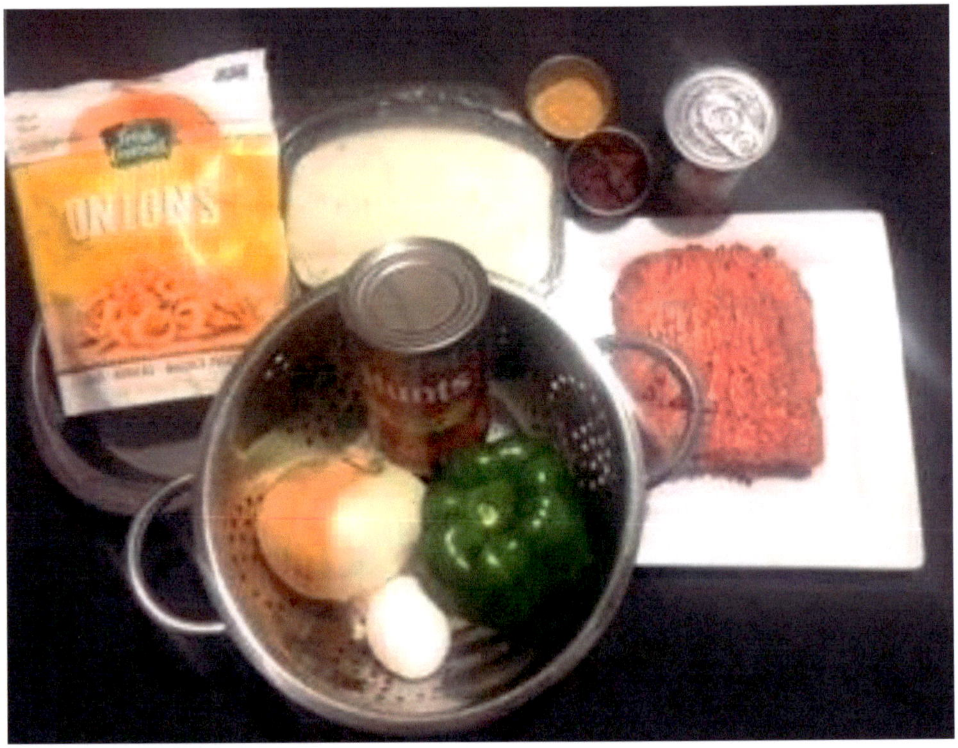

Preheat oven to 350 degrees.

In a bowl, combine the ground meat, egg, chopped onion and bell pepper, seasonings, tomato sauce, and crumpled toast bread. Use your hands to blend all ingredients evenly.

Add even amount of meatloaf mixture into 2 mini cake pans. Since this is a mini cake, the meatloaf will take 45 minutes to an hour.

Once done, allow to cool for approximately 30 minutes.

Use microwave to thaw and heat mashed cauliflower.

After a cooling period, take one of your cake layers out of the pan and place on a plate.

Scoop 3-4 tablespoons of the mashed cauliflower and spread on top of the cake layer. Take the other cake layer out of the pan and place on the top of the first cake layer. Scoop 3-4 tablespoons of the mashed cauliflower and spread evenly across the top like frosting. Then work on spreading the mashed cauliflower around the sides until both layers are fully covered.

Add peas, bacon bits and crispy onions to the top and sides of the cake. My sister even added hot wings to the top her hers. It was a hit!

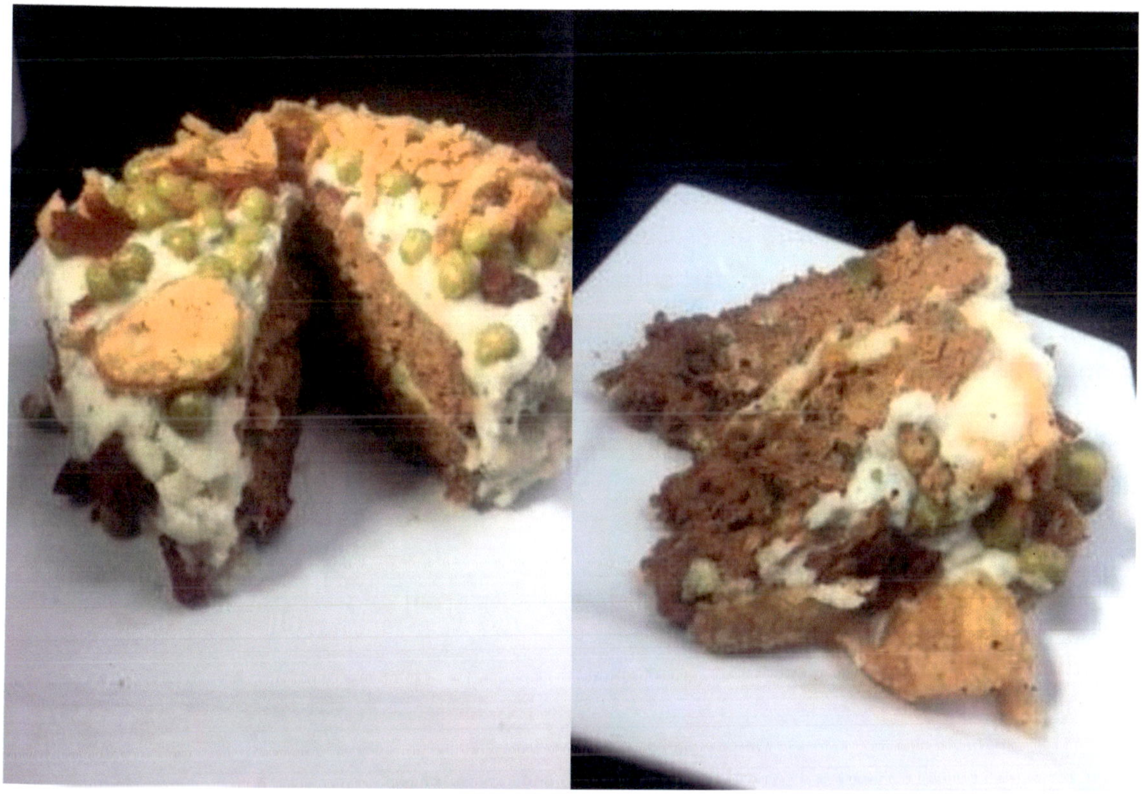

Food For Thought NUMBer 4...

Change is all about mindset. I want all who read this publication to understand making excuses about changing is an obstacle placed by self. It takes the same amount of time to prepare a healthier version of your favorite foods. The cost to eat healthy is also about the same. In some cases, it is more cost efficient. This particular 'Food For Thought' is a must because you have no idea how many make excuses instead of making CHANGE. Diabetes can be deadly. Diabetes can permanently alter your way of living. Please take the time to listen to your body. Be good to your body. I hope the recipe ideas in this book are delicious enough to move those who are diabetics towards CHANGE.

About the Author...

Demitra Bryant was born in Tulsa, Oklahoma and raised in Seattle, Washington. She currently resides in Douglasville, Georgia that is a suburb 15 minutes outside of Atlanta. She is an IT Professional and holds a Bachelor's Degree in Cybersecurity. She also has several Certifications associated with the IT profession. *NUMBers* is Demitra's first publication.

Made in United States
Troutdale, OR
11/03/2026

56844519R00057